Alternative and Complementary Diabetes Care

ALTERNATIVE AND COMPLEMENTARY DIABETES CARE

How to Combine Natural and Traditional Therapies

Diana W. Guthrie, Ph.D., F.A.A.N., C.D.E.

with a History of Diabetes Care
by Richard Guthrie, M.D., F.A.C.E., C.D.E.

John Wiley & Sons, Inc.

New York • Chichester • Weinheim • Brisbane • Singapore • Toronto

Published by John Wiley & Sons, Inc.
Published simultaneously in Canada

Library of Congress Cataloging-in-Publication Data
Guthrie, Diana W.
Alternative and complementary diabetes care : how to combine natural and traditional therapies / Diana W. Guthrie
p. cm.
Includes bibliographical references and index.
ISBN 0-471-34784-1 (paper)
1. Diabetes—Alternative treatment.   I. Title.

RC661.A47 G88 2000
616.4'6206—dc21   99-050258

Printed in the United States of America

10 9 8 7 6 5 4 3 2 1

This book is dedicated to all people who have diabetes;
to Dr. Robert Jackson, my mentor; to Deborah Hinnen and Belinda
Childs, with whom I am fortunate enough to work; and to my
husband, Dr. Richard Guthrie, and our daughters,
Laura, Joyce, and Tammy.

CONTENTS

PREFACE

In 1993, Drs. Eisenberg, Kessler, Foster, Norlock, Calkins, and Delbanco, all respected physicians, published a paper entitled "Unconventional Medicine in the United States." This paper made us aware of the use of alternative and complementary therapies. Dr. Eisenberg and the others noted that over 30 percent of the population in 1993 (over 40 percent in 1997) were using alternative and/or complementary practices, but 71 percent (71.5 percent in 1997) of this population were not sharing this information with their physician.

Various cultures throughout history have identified people who have studied and learned about what heals and what harms (for example, poison plants). Some within these cultures have considered these inquisitors to be a threat, while to others they are saints. However the individuals were labeled, it must be recognized that these people had no special gifts other than a sensitivity to others, to the environment, and, in the case of herbs, a memory that retained varied responses brought about by the use of various herbs. But these skills are present in each one of us. To assist ourselves and others in attaining a healthful life, we just need to take the time to learn and to share our learning.

After completing training and being certified in holistic nursing and healing touch, I wanted to share this knowledge, but when I was asked to write this book, I began to realize what a responsibility it was. Although I was happy to share my knowledge I did not want to be misunderstood. I did not want to lead anyone to do something that was harmful, and most of all, I did not want a person to inappropriately substitute a treatment instead of using a tried-and-true therapy.

It is recognized that there are various approaches to diabetes management that can achieve the same goal of a hemoglobin A_{1c} below 7 percent without the occurrence of significant insulin reactions (low blood sugars). It is also recognized that many of you have not had the opportunity to attend diabetes education classes. With this in mind, Dr. Richard Guthrie has given all of you a short review of diabetes, including an overview of the disease, its potential complications, and general guidelines to expect in the management of Type 1 and Type 2 diabetes. This information should be balanced against the choices made for including any alternative or complementary practices as part of your daily regimen (see appendix A). Therefore, this is not a book to answer all your questions about the use of alternative or complementary care, but it is a resource from which you may choose to make decisions and learn the guidelines for making such decisions.

Information from this book may increase your ability to take better care of yourself. At the least, I hope it will cause you to stop and reflect about whether you are participating in your care as you should. It will assist you in noting whether you are asking the right questions and sharing the right information with your health professional. Working as an informed and educated person will give you, the one with diabetes, better odds of attaining and maintaining a high degree of normalization of blood glucose levels. This has the potential to lead to the reduced risk of developing complications that can be associated with diabetes.

Don't take what you read in this book at face value only. Study and learn for yourself what is best for you or your family member. There are no easy choices. What might work for one person might not work as well for another person, because of differences in metabolic and bodily functions (for example, if you have difficulty absorbing food, you would also have difficulty absorbing an herbal remedy).

Take your time in making decisions and enjoy the possibilities.

Acknowledgments

This book could not have been written without the work of the countless number of other people who have devoted their lives to helping others feel better. I also acknowledge what I have learned from each person who had diabetes and their family members with whom I have had contact. My students have heard this from me many times, "I have never seen any two people have diabetes exactly the same way."

In addition to my husband, Dr. Richard Guthrie, who was a source of untiring support and information about diabetes, I also mention Cathy Feste and Merlene Miller, who have been, probably without their knowing it, guiding lights when I first even thought about writing such a book. Then there is Geri Salis, who was then a pharmacy doctoral student and volunteered her valuable time to hunt up key articles and pertinent references to the material concerning the use of herbs in the field of diabetes mellitus.

Dr. Ronald Hunninghake, one of the physicians at the Center for the Improvement of Human Functioning, in Wichita, Kansas, gave valuable advice and acted as a reviewer for the chapters on vitamins and herbs. His approach to evidence-based medicine along with less traditional individualized treatment has assisted many people to develop a quality of life when many times no hope was given.

Special commendations go to John Gedraitis for his able command of the English language and his editing of the first draft of the manuscript, and to Sharon Buller for her time and energy in preparing the manuscript in its final form.

Joy Pape is another person whom I thank. She gave her energy and talent to the research and writing of the section in chapter 6 on a number of the specific books and their authors' approach to dietary management regimens.

Along with these people, I also mention the tireless work of the American Diabetes Association, the American Association of Diabetes Educators, and the Juvenile Diabetes Foundation, which are all working toward the goals of educating the public and professionals about diabetes and the eradication of this disease.

INTRODUCTION

This book is meant to be a resource that might be used over and over again. You will find the following detailed description of the chapters as a way to guide you in choosing which chapter might be most useful for you at a specific time.

This book is organized in a way that should assist you in remembering what a full, balanced health program should include. This is done by using the acronym PARENT. These letters stand for *Positive thinking*, *Assertiveness*, *Relaxation*, *Exercise*, *Nutrition*, and *Touch* (or *Treatment*). Each of these areas includes various aspects of care and thought that can affect the quality of life that a person who has diabetes might wish to accept, fight, or change. Acceptable daily care activities can be intertwined with those activities that—in your present emotional, physical, mental, or spiritual state—you might wish to improve or change.

Chapter 1 includes an overview of the field of alternative and complementary care. You will learn about some medical schools that are now sensitive to the need to teach future physicians information about the different practices and their pros and cons. It also includes what is being done by the National Center for Complementary and Alternative Medicine at the National Institutes of Health to assist professionals and lay people in recognizing which uses are more scientifically sound and expose other treatments that might not be helpful.

Chapter 2 focuses on thinking positively. Positive thinking helps put things in perspective and leads to a higher immune level and, potentially, to more stable blood glucose levels control. You will learn how positive thinking affects the body from the standpoint of laughter, prayer, reframing, and other choices (for example, meditation, thought stopping, and problem solving). Considerations related to blood sugar control will address logical thinking versus various other approaches to management.

Chapter 3 deals with assertiveness, which is needed for a variety of situations. Dealing with conflict is a part of everyday life in this challenging world. Whether at school, at home, or at work, a person must be able to do what is needed for good health. This chapter contains information on the use of assertiveness in daily life, how to handle conflict, how to develop a win-win approach (negotiation skills), how to handle anger, and how all this relates to blood glucose control.

In Chapter 4 you learn more of what you might already associate with alternative and complementary care—relaxation. You will be reminded of the role relaxation plays in your life and how this affects blood glucose levels directly and indirectly. There are certainly many techniques for learning how to relax. You should find out what works for you. Some of these methods are progressive relaxation, autogenic therapy, deep breathing, imagery, visualization, aroma therapy, and meditation.

Exercise is the focus of chapter 5. You may be a person who would "choose to die" rather than exercise (pain or pleasure), but increasing your activity might be your compromise. Perhaps you could choose to learn Tai chi or yoga as helpful alternatives, or perhaps armchair exercises might be all you could handle. In this chapter, guidance will be given about how to evaluate your present physical condition in relation to safe exercise choices. An evaluation by your health-care professional should be the first step on this path.

Chapter 6 contains information about vitamins and foods, while chapter 7 focuses on herbs. Topics covered include vitamins, minerals, and general reminders on how to become more nutritionally sound, how to lose weight, if needed, and how to keep the weight off, once lost. Aromatherapy will be included. As you will soon learn, aromatherapy includes more than just smelling a pleasant fragrance.

Chapter 8 includes information on such therapies as music therapy and art therapy. It will also include information on specific self-care techniques. Chapter 9 introduces touch and nontouch remedies as well as various therapies that have the potential to lead to improved circulation, improved balance, and an improved sense of well-being. You will find a review of the effect of touch on the body, along with the daily techniques for self-care. Included will be various therapeutic massage practices, therapeutic touch, and the controversy surrounding Reiki and other various energy-based therapies.

Though chapter 10 is the last chapter, it is perhaps the most important. This is where you come in. Your individual choice must be a safe choice that helps and does not hinder the control of your blood glucose levels. This chapter summarizes what you have already read. Most important, it includes the American Diabetes Association guidelines on unproven therapies.

The appendixes that follow include an annotated bibliography, a glossary of terms, useful information on various vitamins and minerals, a listing of herbs that raise or lower blood glucose levels, web sites, and a number of other resources with addresses and phone numbers from which you may obtain more detailed information.

Included in the appendixes is a review of the description and treatment of diabetes mellitus, including methods of monitoring and management. Management methods vary, and what is described is the traditional method that has worked well since its development in the 1930s by Dr. Robert Jackson. This information is included to use as a base of reference for comparing the way the body works and management of diabetes with what is elsewhere in the book.

Be challenged by what you read, but also be careful. Most of all, focus on the goal of having as healthy a life as possible in spite of having diabetes mellitus.

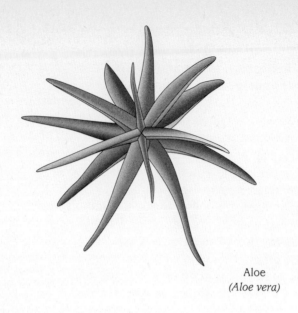

Aloe
(Aloe vera)

1

ALTERNATIVE VERSUS COMPLEMENTARY CARE

Alternative and complementary care practices are increasingly being considered in the field of diabetes. Should they be included as part of the care of people who have diabetes mellitus? Should they both be used? How do the two of these fit together? What use is the acronym PARENT?

THE PARENT APPROACH

Once upon a time, to have a full and healthful self-care program, you needed something to help you remember all the parts of that program. A full stress management or holistic health-care program involves not just diet and exercise. It is also a way of thinking that combines a way of acting, eating, balancing your life, and living life to its fullest. The first letters of the words *Positive* thinking, *Assertiveness, Relaxation, Exercise, Nutrition,* and *Touch* spell the word PARENT. As children, each of us was once nurtured or parented by an adult. Depending on how well you were parented, you learned a variety of things that have become a part of your life as you have become an adult. But as an adult, you now need to be able to parent yourself. The challenge goes on.

These letters can help you remember the overall picture of how to parent yourself. Allow the acronym PARENT to represent the parts of a total self-help or stress management program. Life is filled with stressors (things in the external environment that cause stress). To treat your stress (your responses: physically, emotionally, intellectually, and spiritually) you need a program that incorporates all of these parts.

WHERE TO BEGIN

Alternative and complementary care may be a part of where to begin. As my husband and I say: "You can't reach a goal without starting."

Just as you need a foundation on which to build any structure, you also need a foundation on which you can make more healthful choices. There are lots of choices out there. But having too many choices can be confusing. Which choice is right for me? Will this choice be helpful or harmful?

Looking Backward

> "He conquers who endures." —*Persius*

Ever since diabetes was first recognized, over 2,500 years ago, practitioners and people having the disease have tried to do something to stop it, stabilize it, or cure it. Before the origins of the disease were understood, people thought that chanting incantations or eating certain foods would either prevent it or cure it. Even nowadays, if diagnosed, many people grab at any "cure." Someone might say, "Take this herb; it helped my grandmother." Another might say, "Use this treatment. It made my diabetes go away," while others contend that, "Megadoses of vitamin X keep your blood sugars down."

We now know that either you inherit the disease or something happens directly or indirectly to cause your beta cells in the pancreas not to function or work the way they were supposed to.

Presumably you are receiving the traditional diabetes care from your health practitioner, which requires blood glucose monitoring, meal planning, exercise, medication (for most of you), and stress management (this last part fits more and more frequently into the picture of total management). The nontraditional care you might have chosen might include such things as therapeutic massage, acupuncture, magnets, various doses of vitamins, herbal remedies, and so forth.

Both the media and friends often offer suggestions to try this or use that. How many of you, if you are using anything but the "tried and true," are sharing this information with your health professional without being asked? Perhaps even more important, how many of your health professionals actually know anything about the remedies you are using, or even discount them without knowing if they might help?

You encounter choices about alternative and complementary care in magazines, television and radio ads, and increasingly on the Web. But if you have a chronic illness, then making the choice to use one or more of these remedies can be a potentially dangerous one. How does an herb or vitamin interact with the diabetes medicine you are taking? What happens to blood glucose levels when you perspire profusely or get overheated by sitting in a Jacuzzi? Is this food more beneficial than that food? Is too little fat in the diet as bad as too much fat in the diet? Questions, questions, questions . . . they keep arising, and yet to be safe, you must ask them over and over again.

The Office of Alternative Medicine and Other Programs/Information

Is anything being done to help you make safe and useful choices? In the 1980s, Senator Thomas Harkins of Iowa was suffering from allergies. A variety of traditional health professionals prescribed everything they could to give him some relief. He was at his wits' end when someone suggested that he contact a local holistic practitioner. The therapy recommended by this practitioner relieved his suffering and made his life worthwhile again.

Senator Harkins recognized two things: (1) he found relief through the nontraditional treatment versus the traditional ones and (2) in keeping down health care costs, wasn't it better to prevent disease rather than to wait to get a disease and then treat it?

With the help of other senators, he introduced a bill to Congress that funded the then designated Office of Alternative Medicine (OAM). In the first call for grant proposals to study various remedies—or, as this office termed them, "modalities"—the office was overloaded with the submission of over 450 proposals. Experts in the various fields reviewed these proposals under groupings such as mind/body, energy, nutritionally focused, and so forth. The initial funding for these studies also lead to the formation of centers for the study of alternative and complementary care. The University of Texas for cancer; Columbia University's College of Physicians and Surgeons for women's health; the Kessler Institute for Rehabilitation for stroke and neuro-rehabilitation; Bastyr University for HIV and AIDS; the University of Virginia School of Nursing and the University of Maryland School of Medicine for pain; Stanford University for aging; Minneapolis Medical Research Center for Addictions; Beth Israel Hospital and Harvard Medical School for internal medicine; the University of California at Davis for asthma and allergy; and the Palmer College of Chiropractic for chiropractic care are some of the earliest funded programs. In 1999 the OAM became the National Center for Complementary and Alternative Medicine (CAM). In 1999 Capital University, in Washington, D.C., graduated for the first time medical health professionals who had attended a two-year course in alternative and complementary care—or integrative medicine. Plans are underway to make such a program available to physicians in the Midwest and western parts of the United States.

To date, over 50 percent of the 127 medical schools in the country are now offering required or elective courses on alternative and complementary medicine. These schools are addressing not only what needs to be studied but also what resources are available to help answer the questions of clients. Many more physicians are obtaining extra training so that they are able to choose from a variety of remedies (or modalities) to best meet the needs of their patients. When asked in a survey, more than 80 percent of medical students indicated they would like further training in Complementary and Alternative Medicine (CAM). As of this writing, one-third of family practice residencies already provide some type of CAM education.

Recommendations and Resources

As a health-care consumer you should know what the health-care experts are recommending. The following recommendations were made in 1996 by a panel of experts representing the American Medical Association, the American Academy of Family Practice, the American Association of Medical Colleges, the American Medical Students' Association, and other organizations: (1) medical and nursing education should include information about complementary practices; (2) medical and nursing education about each complementary and alternative practice should include information about the history of the remedy, its scientific foundation, the educational preparation needed to give or recommend a remedy, evidence of safety, being certified or licensed by a qualified organization; and (3) national centers of excellence should continue to be developed to foster cooperation among complementary practitioners, nurses, physicians, and to promote a smoother flow of information among education, research, and clinical practice.

More information appears daily. Web sites offer more and more choices, and it's up to you to judge whether the information is helpful or not. The National Diabetes Information Clearinghouse has a search line you may request: Complementary and Alternative Therapies for Treatment of Diabetes Mellitus (see appendix F). This is an annotated bibliography about articles that have appeared in lay publications. New journals have been published, including *Alternative and Complementary Medicine, Alternative Therapies in Health and Medicine, Advances in Medicine,* and the *International Journal for Subtle Energy.*

A nurse may be certified in aromatherapy and in holistic nursing. Lay people and health professionals may be certified in healing touch or become Reiki masters. Training is available to study acupuncture and become certified. Naturopathy and homeopathy are fields that have reawakened interest. But this is just the surface, because many people want to know more, especially about energy and healing.

The summer (1997) issue of *Alternative Health Practitioner* focused on "integrated" centers—those centers that combine traditional with nontraditional care by making available physical facilities, developing plans with individual patients, and educating patients in the use of helpful remedies. Recognized universities, such as Harvard and Yale, are offering courses, some nationwide, on alternative and complementary health-care practices. These are attended by health professionals, by clergy, and by people such as you.

There is now a *Physicians' Desk Reference* for herbal medicine help line (888-859-8053). "Herbal Remedies in the Pharmacy," an article in the July 1997 issue of *U.S. Pharmacist,* has concluded that since herbal remedies are gaining in popularity, pharmacists need to know how to counsel patients.

More than four hundred herbs have been found to lower blood sugar levels. Only a small number of these, in proportion to what is possibly available, have been evaluated scientifically.

In the November/December issue (1997) of *Practical Diabetes International,* an article appeared on the "Prevalence of Complementary Medicine Usage within a Diabetes Clinic." Authors recognized its use and shared how the use of complementary medicine may have effects on the management of diabetes in the United Kingdom.

As of 1994, herbs, minerals, and vitamins (also termed phytomedicinals or neutraceuticals) can be sold as dietary supplements. The Dietary Supplement Health and Education Act (DSHEA)(1994) specifies that to qualify for this "category," no therapeutic claims can appear on any label. The label must also note that the product has not been reviewed by the Food and Drug Administration. As part of this DSHEA, the president appointed a new commission comprised of leaders in the field of herbal medicine. They are charged to amass information in order to guide the future process of labeling and handling these products.

CONCERNS AND CAUTIONS

Of increasing importance is the ongoing research to help us understand the role of the immune system and its association with the ability to get infections. It has been found that an overactive immune system as well as an underactive immune system can both lead to problems. An overactive immune system might attack itself (for example, autoimmune diseases such as Type 1 diabetes; allergies; rheumatoid arthritis; ulcerative colitis). An underactive immune system leads to frequent infections, so you must take great care in what treatment you choose to use or to not use. This is especially important when choosing herbal remedies.

Certain herbs have been identified, through existing evidence, not to be safe (either by specific action or potential for incorrect use), and they should be used only under the directions of a qualified professional. They are listed below for emphasis and will be discussed again in the chapter on herbs (chapter 7). Based on references dated from 1993 to 1997, the following herbs are considered unsafe: chaparral (*Larrea tridentata*) as it can lead to liver damage; ephedra (also known as mahuang or *Ephedra sinica*) should not be used if someone is taking an MAO inhibitor (monoamine oxidase, which is found in some antidepressants), or if heart disease, diabetes, or high blood pressure is present. Hydrangea (*Hydrangea arborescens*) can be problematic, depending on the choice of the source. The correct source is the root, but using the leaves can lead to a severe problem, as the leaves contain cyanide. Poke root (*Phytolacca decantra*) may be fatal in children and results in vomiting. Sassafras (*Sassafras albidum*) though an old-time, springtime remedy, contains a carcinogen (a chemical capable of causing cancer) and is also known to cause liver damage. Yohimbine (*Corynanthe yohimbe*) can cause high blood pressure and anxiety. This herb should not be used if a person has kidney disease or a mental illness.

Note that moderately unsafe herbs are considered to be bearberry (not recommended for use in acute inflammation, pregnancy, or for prostate disorders), or black/blue cohosh (should not be used during pregnancy or for anyone having a chronic disease such as diabetes). A large dose of boneset is toxic. Liver damage can be caused by comfrey. Juniper should not be used during pregnancy and is known to cause kidney disease if used too long. Licorice should not be used if a person is pregnant or has diabetes, heart disease, or high blood pressure. Lobelia has a nicotinelike effect and should not be used in pregnancy. If used it should be given in doses of less than 50 mg/day and only for a short time. Wormwood should not be used during pregnancy.

On the other hand, in *American Druggist,* April 1997, a physician promotes that diabetes patients can benefit from certain supplements. The doctor felt that primrose oil, which contains gamma-linolenic acid (GLA), taurine (which thins the blood), vitamin E, and magnesium (which can increase insulin sensitivity), would be useful for people who have diabetes. Reputable scientific journals are the sources for his claims.

The chapter on diabetes in *Alternative Medicine: The Definitive Guide* compiled by the Burton Goldberg Group explains the disease and then follows with recommendations for treatment. It includes references from the work of James Anderson, a physician from the Department of Veterans Affairs at the University of Kentucky in Lexington, speaking on complex fibers and complex carbohydrates, and Dr. Jonathan Wright, director of the Tahoma Clinic I, Kent, Washington, who presents guidelines for people with diabetes.

What they say sounds familiar:

- Eliminate concentrated, refined sugar and sugar products.
- Avoid junk foods.
- Eat whole grains, fresh fruits and vegetables; reduce or eliminate stimulants; eat a small amount of protein in snacks; and take off excess weight.

The diet chapter discusses food intolerances and nutritional supplements, such as the B, C, and E vitamins, and the minerals, magnesium, potassium, chromium, and zinc, plus coenzyme (CoQ_{10}), amino acids, and the digestive enzymes. Credible references are included.

Dr. Andrew Weil, in another resource, advises that rest provides a boost for the immune system, along with eating whole foods, less protein, more carbohydrate foods, such as vegetables, fruits, and grains, and less fat. He states that the following natural substances boost the immune system. These are shiitake or reishi mushrooms, echinacea (this will be discussed in detail later) or astragalus, vitamin C, vitamin E, selenium, alpha- and beta-carotenes, CoQ_{10}, and B complex vitamins (people with Type 2 diabetes should be careful of the amount of B_3 or niacin the product contains). These have been found to block chemical reactions and neutralize free radicals that cause tissue damage. He also recommends maintaining good oral health and exercising almost daily.

But there will still be disagreements among credible people and sound scientific references, especially in this field. What about antibiotics killing good bacteria with the bad? An *American Druggist* 1997 article makes a case for the indiscriminate use of antibiotics when they aren't really needed. Physicians are recognizing (and now being taught) that antibiotics should be used only for specific purposes. They are also learning about how to replace good bacteria through the use of lactobacillus tablets or drinking acidophilus milk (which you can buy from a grocer). If the good bacteria are killed, then the yeast growth can rise rapidly, and you end up with a yeast infection or worse. Acidophilus keeps yeast under control, helps digestion, and supplies B vitamins.

Sheila Hunter is a pharmacist who is the author of a home study course on nontraditional medication, homeopathy, and herbal medicine. Besides describing the field, her course on homeopathy gives a listing of some of the signs and symptoms a person might report and the corresponding remedies that might be used. Each group of remedies includes alternatives, but not dosages. It reports the need to look for color of the skin and/or eyes, to feel general or specific areas of the body, to locate discomfort, to note the time of day the symptoms are worse, the person's mood, and so on. It includes summaries on the most frequently used homeopathic remedies. The herbal section includes a description and explanation of a variety of uses of specific herbs as well.

Good, careful studies can give much useful information rather than be looked at as "taking away" the "herb I want to use." In India, for instance, researchers studied guar gum and other herbs and compared them to conventional diabetes medication. In this instance, they found that the herb was useful as an adjunct to therapy or as complementary to the traditional therapy they were using. It made a good treatment even better. In this particular study, they also found some herbs, when used in a certain way, had a better effect on lowering the blood sugar than the standard treatment. These may be the origins of new medications once they have undergone other tests. Studying these herbs has the potential of bringing about the discovery of more effective medicines.

What Is "Natural"

Since herbs are considered natural, you often read or hear the statement, "If it's natural, it has to be safe." But this is not necessarily so. The term "natural" in the United States means that the product does not contain slaughterhouse byproducts or petrochemical derivatives. It also means that the product is made up of mainly botanicals (things from earth pigments). The European criteria for something termed "natural" include the information that the product must: support the natural functions of the skin, the active ingredients must be natural (from the earth), no testing can have been done on animals or obtained in any way cruel to animals, must fulfill the legal requirements, must be environmentally sound, and must be biodegradable in a short period of time.

Special Care

You should be aware of the "worst case scenario," such as a person who has Type 1 diabetes stopping insulin while using a certain remedy. This is a clear cause for concern. The claims of certain remedies to improve diabetes might be helpful only as long as the principles are maintained. For example, the major principle would be to normalize blood glucose levels the majority of the time, with few below normal blood sugar episodes experienced. If the rest of the body is not harmed, the use of the complementary therapy would really be a blessing. An alternative therapy such as exercising after meals, rather than continued eating, would clearly be beneficial.

It is possible that some unusual practices could be indirectly effective. If you "tied some coral to your arm" or "drank milk that had pearls boiled in it"—practices suggested by an Indian healer—you might be more aware of your activity and food intake to the point where your blood sugars did improve. This could be due to your increased awareness of doing something believed to be helpful that in itself might not necessarily be so. Therefore, your use of a product may not result directly in blood glucose levels decreasing but indirectly, by the awareness you have of controlled caloric intake and use of a product in relation to what you usually eat to feel satisfied. Various models of practice, in this way, could actually offer some support to attaining the goal of normal glucose levels.

MODELS OF PRACTICE

There are many other practices of which you should be aware.

The allopathic model is the traditional model, which focuses on medicine and surgery.

The Piman model might include an allopathic physician or nurse, but more often a shaman or herbalist who assists in getting rid of impurities of the body and upholding spiritual needs.

The Curanderismo model often includes an herbalist or a medium. This model works with individuals or groups and provides them a specific regimen to follow to restore balance.

The Chinese programs could include a physician, a shaman, an herbalist or a masseur, as all address the concerns of energy blockages in the body and the balance of the yin versus the yang (that is, male versus female; hot versus cold, etc.).

The homeopathy model looks at the essence or history and can then suggest diluted solutions to mimic the illness but at a much lower strength, so that the body's immune system responds, as it might with a vaccination.

The chiropractic model studies bones and specifically the nerves of various parts of the body. This is said to complement allopathic treatments by adjusting or balancing the person's body so that the individual would respond better to the treatment or medicine given.

The naturopathic model uses the herbs and vitamins of a balanced diet as well as supplements when needed. Supplements may be helpful for healing but not necessarily curing.

Culture and Beliefs

A study about Mexican Americans of Hispanic origin found that 17 percent of patients reported using herbs to treat their diabetes. This needs to be taken into consideration by health professionals working with this or any other specific culture. Their religious and spiritual beliefs are also important to consider. You may be one of this group (78 percent in this particular population) that believes it is God's will for you have diabetes. If this is your belief, it should be honored as should any other beliefs that do not hurt or harm yourself or others.

Cultural norms will influence an individual's response to having diabetes in that culture. If you have a headache, the healer treats it. For Tongans, who are Polynesian, the massage of the head by a foot might be the solution. If that doesn't work, then it might be thought to be due to a spiritual cause. If your headache was due to low blood glucose levels, unless your health-care worker cooperated with what the healer was doing and vice versa, it might be possible for you to suffer from problems that would result from an even lower blood sugar.

African-Americans and others enjoy "spiritualcise"—a mind-body exercise program that includes low-impact aerobic movement, gospel music, and a forum for discussion.

Programs that originate in various cultures could be useful to assist people from other populations. Sharing information helps all people with diabetes to live a better life.

Healing versus Curing

Just to set the record straight, healing is not curing, but curing is certainly healing. Healing is described as rebalancing the body so that curing (when the body moves from an ill state to a well state) might occur. Healing might occur only spiritually or emotionally or mentally rather than physically. Many energy therapies are based on healing rather than curing. For example, healing practices might sooth the pain, but the illness doesn't go away.

A more recognizable example of healing is when hypnosis is used to help people in pain imagine that their few minutes of comfort actually seem like hours of comfort.

In Lourdes, France, a person might be healed (feel better in mind or mind and body) or be cured—get up and walk. This healing may have a holistic effect or just an effect on being able to miraculously walk. (A team of doctors and priests determines if the "walking" was truly a miracle or not.)

WHERE TO START

"A journey of a thousand miles begins with a single step."
—*A Chinese proverb*

"The ultimate measure of a man (a woman) is not where he (she) stands in moments of comfort and convenience, it is where he (she) stands at times of challenge and controversy."
—*Dr. Martin Luther King Jr.*

All parts of the body (including genetics), mind (includes perceptions, intelligence), emotions, and beliefs (spirituality) are involved in holistic interventions. This is why the initials of the PARENT approach should get you back to the initial purpose of this book, which is to give you resources from which to obtain further information and from which the most appropriate decisions might be made. This should take into account the unique needs of your total being.

The results of any or all of these interventions have the potential to help or to harm. If wise choices are made, the potential is an increased quality of life for many people and a potentially increasing basis for the prevention of disease in spite of having diabetes.

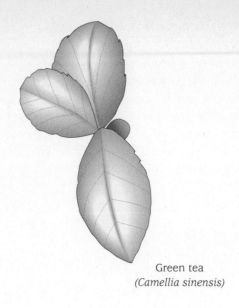

Green tea
(Camellia sinensis)

2

PUTTING THINGS STRAIGHT

"Opportunity . . . often, it comes disguised in the form of misfortune or temporary defeat." —*Carl Jung*

Every time Edward entered a room, his family stopped talking. He thought it was all just in his mind, but this occurred over and over again. He had been diagnosed as having diabetes just a few months earlier. This did not happen before his diagnosis, or not that he noticed.

During therapy sessions, Edward became more confident as he recognized that he had a chronic disease he could control. He learned to reframe the "talking that stopped" as really concern that these people had for him. Now he feels pleased when he hears the talking stop when he enters a room. He says to himself it is because he is special enough that they wish him not to see their concern. This recognition has now turned into an opportunity to educate his family.

POSITIVE THINKING

"If you can dream it, you can do it." —*Walt Disney*

"To look up is joy." —*Confucius*

Positive thinking is the ability to change or reformulate thinking so that you emphasize the upside instead of the downside in life. You think positively when you are buying a gift for a loved one instead of begrudging the money spent. You think positively when you choose to smile rather than frown at a passerby.

An appropriate example of positive thinking is to focus on the good aspects of having diabetes mellitus. This should not negate diabetes as a terribly threatening disease, but there are some good things that can come from bad things. Positive thinking assists you in putting things straight. You can think about the positives in having diabetes rather than trying to escape the fact that you have diabetes. You are on a voyage of discovery. Positive thinking aids you in looking at your life with new eyes and reframing the negative as the positive.

Your "new eyes" might have an effect on how you are now caring for yourself. You might be making more appropriate choices about the foods you eat, the exercise you do, or the quiet times you choose to take during the day. You might find yourself healthier than you were before the diagnosis of diabetes, in that you have fewer colds and sore throats because your blood glucose levels are normal more of the time and you know more about better self-care.

As you read, you will find ways to assist yourself to became a more positive thinker in addition to learning more about affirmations and attitude, reframing, thought stopping, time management, laughter, and prayer. You truly are on a voyage of discovery—a voyage of discovery about yourself.

Attitude

If you don't have a good attitude, you have started out on the wrong foot. A favorite saying I share is "I'm okay, 'cause God don't make no junk." This line was on a poster depicting a disheveled child who has dirt on his face but a twinkle in his eye. Having a positive attitude is the right way to start, just as accepting that you have diabetes is the best attitude to have when working with your health professional.

If you have a "bad" attitude, you won't see the worth in doing anything. You will be resistant to learning about the disease and how to care for yourself. You will be less cooperative when a health professional or family member supports you in learning self-care techniques. You will see little worth in prolonging life in a healthful way. In denying your state of health, you ignore diabetes rather than allowing diabetes to be an opportunity rather than an obstacle.

With a positive attitude, you become willing to listen. You are willing to learn. You are willing to take that next step beyond recognition that you have the disease. Surely no one wants to have diabetes. But with acceptance of the fact that you or your loved one has diabetes, you are now able to take into account the various pieces of information and techniques that can help you redevelop a good quality of life for yourself. One of these first pieces of information is in the conscious or subconscious stating of positive affirmations.

Affirmations

Affirmations can be both negative and positive. A positive or negative affirmation can influence your attitude about anything. Saying "I choose to have fruit for dessert" rather than "I *have* to have fruit for dessert" represents a positive way of affirming rather than being negative. (Reframing will be discussed later in this chapter as a way of changing a negative into a positive.)

How can you use positive affirmations? Emile Coué was known to say, "Every day, and in every way, I am becoming better and better." He is known for his research in positive thinking. He found, as did others, that a person who thinks positively is ill less frequently than a person who thinks negatively. Therefore, a person can state a positive affirmation, such as "I choose to take good care of myself because I'm worth it."

The opposite is also true. If this is said frequently enough, it will be believed, just as if you tell yourself you are no good, eventually you will actually believe that you are not good. As you choose to make more appropriate choices, tell yourself, "Pretty soon that choice I made will be the choice that will become a part of me."

When you take the path of affirming yourself, you can choose to help yourself in a variety of ways. You could purchase a poster that reflects what you are wishing to affirm to yourself. You could take three-by-five-inch index cards and write out your affirmative statements and then post these cards all over the house so that every time you turn around, you are faced with a positive statement.

This technique has been very useful for individuals who have problems with overeating. If you are one of these people, you could put a card right on the refrigerator door. It would remind you to believe what you wrote on the card. The affirmative statement reaffirms your choice not to eat something unhealthful at this time.

Other resources that you can use are dictating devices that can be placed on key chains, or carried in a pocket or purse. (They are advertised as being able to help you to locate your car. You state into the microphone, before leaving the site of the car, some identifying characteristics that help you remember where you parked.) You could use this same device to state positively who you now believe you are or whatever other affirmative statement you wish to repeat, and you'll be able to hear this message just by pressing a button. You could also leave a message on your answering machine so that later, when you go to retrieve your messages, you will hear your own voice reminding you that you are feeling and thinking positively about yourself.

OTHER TECHNIQUES

There are a number of other techniques that may be self-taught.

Reframing

> "People are just about as happy as they make up their minds to be." —*Abraham Lincoln*

> "It all depends on how we look at things and not on how they are themselves." —*Carl Jung*

We mentioned the word *reframing*. Did you know that you can reframe almost anything that is a negative to a positive? A person recently was told that she needed to start dialysis to flush out the waste products in her body, since her own kidneys were no longer able to do this job. Needless to say, it was very difficult for her to find any kind of affirmation about this. But she found one by Wayne Dyer, stating, "I am not my body." In other words, although her body was failing, her body was not her mind or soul. She could still think, talk, feel, love, and laugh. She stated, "I can feel good about myself in spite of losing the working ability of my kidneys, since I recognize that my body is not my mind."

Put success in your life by reframing and using positive affirmations. Although some people seem to have more success than others, success can be built into problem solving and everyday life.

Reframe negative thoughts. Allow yourself to grieve, but don't get stuck with grieving. For example, when something bad happens, it's your choice if you let that episode ruin your whole life. As mentioned before, but in a different way, allow obstacles to become opportunities. You can take part in fixing a problem even if you didn't cause it. You didn't cause your diabetes, but you surely can do things to help integrate self-care needs into your daily lifestyle.

If you develop a healthy attitude, even the most boring task of self-care can be perceived as a step toward a greater goal.

When a negative enters your life, find its positive counterpart. Say it over and over again, as an affirmation, until you develop some ownership of the statement. Give yourself this choice of saying something in a different way that will have more positive meaning in your life.

Perhaps you think you are too busy to take the time to reframe a thought or to redo an action that could have been harmful into something that would be helpful. Are you one of those people who has said, "I don't have time to do my blood sugar test"? Do you recognize that now there is a machine that can test your blood sugar in fifteen seconds or less? It only takes a few seconds more to wash your hands and get out the supplies before administering the test. Just as these machines can now offer test results in an even shorter time, so can you take time to develop a reframe that can give you the results you need.

It is true that self-care techniques require time. Taking time away from other activities or having the time to participate in self-care can be frustrating. As part of reframing, a person could use another technique, called time management.

Time Management

Time, as described by John Cabot Zinn, is too often a prison. To aid yourself, he recommends that you look at time as a product of thought. He also recommends that you live in the present, meditate or have some quiet time each day, and simplify your life as much as possible.

Time management is a way to simplify your life by organizing your activities and thoughts so that all the important things in your life may be accomplished. It takes anywhere from ten to thirty minutes at the beginning of the week, and only one to ten minutes a day.

You can develop your own method of managing your time. For instance, you could wake up in the morning, and before you even get out of bed, think of the things you must accomplish during the day. Which of these items is most important to accomplish? What next? and so forth.

Is there an item that you would rather not do, like testing your blood for sugar? Immediately think what positive thing you would do if your blood sugar was in the normal range. What about if it were quite high? Your reframe could be, "I'm grateful that I know whom to call or what to do when my blood sugar is this high." Your attitude could be, "I'd rather know and be able to do something about it than let problems creep up on me and really become ill." Your affirmation might then be, "I am worth caring for, therefore, I choose to do those things that would best help me."

A weekly assessment leads you to determine what you need to accomplish by the end of the seven days. It takes a little longer, in most instances, for it often involves coordinating your schedule with some other person's, or the rest of the family's schedule. You might have a doctor's appointment that conflicts with a special day or a previous commitment. The time it might take to alter one or more of the activities usually takes a little longer than not planning and unknowingly adding a number of unnecessary errands. By planning for the changes you make, these other alterations in the schedule allow you more effective use of your time.

Time management could also involve the ABC's. *A* would stand for ASAP (as soon as possible); *B* could stand for "before the end of the day" or "before the end of the week" or "before the end of the month." *C* is the "can wait" pile. This last pile has a tendency to get higher and higher—so plan to reduce it once every three to six months so you aren't overwhelmed by the anticipation of reducing the effort. Remember, you can reduce this pile by noting whether you really need to do that item or whether you might be able to assign that item to another person.

Thought Stopping

What if you want to stop your thinking? Thought stopping is too often a difficult thing to do. But thought stopping is a useful tool. It has been found that if you forcefully try to stop your thoughts, your thoughts appear to be more resistant and seem to be more difficult to stop. It's similar to what happens when you consciously try to sleep or relax. The outcome is usually that you become more wide awake, or more tense, or think more rather than less. The following are some techniques for helping to stop your thoughts:

If you wake up in the middle of the night and write down your thoughts, then you will find you are better able to drop back into a sleep state. If you are in the middle of a meeting or driving along the road and a thought comes into your mind so that you can't keep your focus on the meeting or on your driving, take a second to write down the thought (or dictate it). So, keep that pad and pencil or recorder handy.

You can visualize putting your thoughts in a bubble, in a drawer, or in a box at the time you wish to "thought stop." This is not so that the thoughts will be forgotten, but so that you can choose, at that time, to keep your mind on something else. This is a technique that is often taught to people who learn to meditate. You must have as clear a mind as possible to be able to meditate effectively, whether it be for a few minutes or longer. Using one of these techniques will aid in clearing your mind so that you may more successfully reach a state of quietness and calmness.

Journaling

> "You can if you think you can." —*George Reeves* (sixth-grade
> teacher of Norman Vincent Peale)

Journaling is also useful, as is talking to a friend, or counselor or pastor. When journaling, you are writing to yourself, so you can dictate or write any thoughts or concerns of the moment. You are free to say what you please and do not have to worry about how you say it or what you write.

Use journaling for problem solving. Act as your own therapist by working yourself through a problem or situation. Ask yourself questions and then answer them. It is safe to write or state your feelings in this way, especially if you are angry about someone or something. Often, the situation does not look as bad, once you have used this tool of communication.

Be quiet for a few minutes before you start, or jump right in. Dating your journal entries will help to put things into perspective if you later choose to review what you previously said or wrote. Let your intuition lead you to what you write or dictate. Note observations. Remember dialogue. Write a letter. Describe the scene or the person.

Participate in a technique called "free association." Start with a word or phrase and let your mind wander freely as to what to put down or speak next. Don't worry about style—and finish with a prayer or quiet moment.

SUBTLE ENERGY

What is subtle energy? Have you ever tried to push the same poles of a magnet together? You can't see anything there, but there is a resistance or subtle energy that keeps these two ends apart. Japanese researchers have used magnet therapy for years to treat chronic fatigue syndrome, which they believe is the result of an energy deficiency that magnetic fields seem to correct.

Whether the effect of magnets is a placebo (or false) effect or not, people who use them have experienced decreased pain and depression. Studies are now being done on the use of magnets to determine what cannot be explained by any other cause. We'll talk a little more about electromagnetic fields in chapter 8—but for now, note that electromagnetic field therapy is now approved by the FDA for the treatment of bone fractures that have a problem healing.

Your surroundings provide a subtle energy that can have an effect on your ability to think positively. If you live in a cluttered place and feel comfortable about it, no further word is needed. If you feel that your surroundings are filled with extra and unnecessary items, then your should consider Feng shui.

Feng shui (pronounced "fung schway") literally means "wind and water." This is the Chinese art of placement. It has been practiced for thousands of years to promote harmony and balance between humans and the environment or nature. Feng shui espouses that even the color or placement of your furniture can affect your health, finances, and relationships (that is, subtle energy).

You can study this field or contact a consultant, Valerie Dow (316-788-3676) who can assist you in arranging your own furniture, especially in your sleeping quarters. With an adequately spaced, colored, and designed environment, you should awaken refreshed.

For a better start of the day, take deep breaths and allow yourself to relax and become aware of how the room around you feels. Is noise pollution a problem? Does the air smell the way you feel most comfortable? Is there lack of clutter? What about electrical and magnetic fields? We're learning more about them, from the type of alarm clock next to your bed to electric blankets (only if left plugged in while you are sleeping).

Finally, consider radiation. You can actually buy a kit from a hardware store to check the radiation from your microwave and determine if the levels are low enough. This is another example of subtle energy. Subtle energy is present in a variety of ways and can affect your sense of space, loss, or connectedness.

Avatar

Avatar is the name of a course that is based on the premise that your beliefs will cause you "to create or attract situations and events that you experience as you live." The purpose of this course is to assist you in exploring your own belief system and to teach you tools to change what you wish to change. You learn how to expand the awareness of your beliefs and how they affect your life, to enhance this awareness, and to explore the foundation of the beliefs while learning the techniques to assist in altering the thinking and action responses to those beliefs. Other higher levels of training are also offered (407-788-3090).

Laughter

The other side of the quiet, reflective therapy is laughter. Laughter, like prayer, has been studied and been found to be associated with the release of endorphins, much like exercise. In fact, laughter *is* exercise (the pleasant kind).

Laughter not only relieves depression, but it also increases the sense of well-being, as any exercise program will tend to do. It influences positive thinking as well as the work of helper T cells (the cells that help to prevent infection), and thus has an affect on fighting disease.

While humor may not actually have been tested for its effect on lowering blood glucose levels, it has been noted by Nancy Brooks, a sociologist, and others to be helpful in "lightening up" the impact of chronic illness or disability. Nancy and her co-researchers found there seems to be less laughter the longer a person has a disease, especially if the condition has worsened over time. This result appears to be not from the disease itself, but from the people involved, who think that their condition is not a laughing matter. When these individuals are given "permission" to laugh, it appears to help the whole family in addition to the one who has the disease or chronic disability. (The people who participated in the study had diabetes or multiple sclerosis or rheumatoid arthritis.)

Garrison Keillor says, "Humor is not a trick. Humor is a presence in the world, . . . like grace . . . and shines on everybody." Hopefully, humor was a part of your diabetes education. Of course, I don't mean an actual course on humor, but a program similar to one found in the Diabetes Treatment and Research Center in Wichita, Kansas. On "graduation," the diabetes educators often walk into the classroom with masks or other silly objects on their heads or faces. The participants break out into laughter, as do we all.

The first joke I saw about diabetes, long before blood glucose meters were available, was a drawing of a hospitalized patient with a sugar container on its side on a hospital bedside table. The accompanying caption read, "Mr. Brown, I see that you're spilling sugar again."

There is an old Japanese proverb, "Time spent laughing is time spent with the gods." At a midwestern diabetes camp, the boys and girls look forward to the education sessions, which combine laughter with learning through the use of puppets, games, and role-playing.

After the most serious occurrence, there is always someone who can find the humor in it. But humor can also be cruel. If humor involves teasing, chances are it will hurt. If a person becomes the focus of a joke and the joke is about an embarrassing situation, feelings will be hurt. Humor can be dangerous if its focus is away from aiding self-esteem.

Do you have a book of jokes to read when things get "too heavy"? Perhaps, like Norman Cousins, the author of *Anatomy of an Illness,* you view videos that give you a chuckle or a full belly laugh. You might collect things that bring out a smile or a laugh, place them in an accessible box, and pull them out when things seem the worst. Get some silly things to put on and wear them at the right time. Have an attitude of playfulness. Read Loretta LaRoche's book *Relax: You May Only Have a Few Minutes Left: Using the Power of Humor to Overcome Stress in Your Life and Work* (1998).

Another of Norman Cousins' books is a useful resource. He explains how laughter benefits your body in *Head First: The Biology of Hope and the Healing Power of the Human Spirit.*

If the air is tense, tell a funny experience about yourself: like the time I returned to a restaurant to get a receipt I'd forgotten. In front of the restaurant was a fire truck, a number of police cars, and my friend, who was walking out of the building carrying a little black box, one of the first cases used to carry a blood sugar monitor. He had mistakenly left this on the floor by his chair.

You guessed it. They thought it was a bomb until my friend, who had also returned to retrieve it, relieved their curiosity.

Laughter is healing when it is effectively used. When you laugh you decrease the cells that make you sick by increasing the power of your immune system. Laughter also releases subtle energy that is "contagious" to those in your presence. Positive thinking and any of its parts, a few of which we have discussed in this chapter, have an effect on the subtle energy that is within you and around you. The pain, fatigue, or depression you experience may be subtly altered when your blood glucose levels are too high or too low.

Spirituality

Spirituality is influenced by a variety of energy factors, including exercise, and may, in fact, result in a subtle energy flow. In this chapter, spirituality will focus more on relations, beliefs, and faith, although subtle energy must also be taken into account. (See chapters 8 and 9 for more information about this area.)

Spirituality is our relationship with the eternal and the universal or internal. Spirituality is an integral part of being human. Spirituality involves subtle energy. It involves one's self, relationships with others, creative expression, familiar rituals, and religious practices. It gives meaning to life and thought as they relate to a higher power, illness, and death. Spirituality is part of the balance of life and can help you feel in control of your diabetes management. Health professionals may be on-call twenty-four hours a day, but they are not always there when you need to make a decision. Consideration must be given and energy spent to include your mental, physical, emotional, and spiritual sides in relation to your diabetes management, your social and daily activities, and response to treatment.

Spirituality and diabetes relate to a loss of ability to do things in the way you did before being diagnosed. The diagnosis of diabetes may have altered the meaning and purpose of your life. You are now, if you have not already done so, looking for the interconnections that can be found by recognizing that the changes made in your life are stressful, that what you choose to do or not do might make you feel guilty. You have also lost a sense of connectedness. Health-care providers might make you feel more guilty or give you guidance on how to make better choices. If you have not done so already, note how your illness might interfere with your life goals. Are you motivated to achieve your goals in spite of having diabetes? Do you know, or have you recognized, what is most important to you and how this brings you strength? What gives your life meaning? Contact Dr. Susan Rush Michael for a copy of her spiritual assessment tool. (E-mail: Susanm@nevada.edu) Spirituality is an important part of your life. Assess your own needs and determine how they might assist you as you progress through life.

Ninety-nine percent of family doctors felt that religious beliefs and practices, such as prayer, could aid in healing. Eighty percent of these health professionals thought that relaxation or meditation techniques should be a part of doctors' training. Other studies have shown that 83 percent of women believe faith can help someone who is recovering from illness, or has actually aided in healing. Forty percent of hospitalized patients say their religious faith is the most important fact that enables them to cope. For example, those who attend religious services at least once a week have stronger immune systems. Over a twenty-eight-year period of study, the risk of dying was 25 percent less in men and 35 percent less in women if they attended religious services frequently (taking into account their health practices, social ties, and well-being). If prayed for, patients had fewer complications when admitted to an intensive-care setting.

Hospitalization stays are two and a half times longer for older patients who do not have a religious affiliation. And older patients are less likely to be hospitalized if they regularly attend religious services. In an older study, it was revealed that patients assigned a daily chaplain visit had shorter hospital stays, used less nurse time, and took fewer pain medications—so if you're hospitalized, don't forget to let your religious affiliation know or check in with the hospital chaplain.

Spiritual assistance through prayer is now being recognized by third-party payers. The HIP Health Plan of New York, is the first managed care organization to provide financial reimbursement for spiritual assistance through intervention by trained hospital pastors and chaplains.

Meditation

Meditation allows you to reach a calm and relaxed mental state. To reach this state, you need to block out the environment around you. This is not a forced process but one that allows you to focus on a sound, a thought, a picture or vision, or just on a spot on the wall.

You must be positively focused. You can attain this state through sitting quietly and centering on your breathing. You can use prayer to attain this state, utilizing a contemplative type of prayer.

I had an experience with meditation I will never forget. I was learning about one Native American tribe's way of mediation where you sit facing each direction for a non-designated period of time: east, south, west, and north. As you faced each direction you observed your surroundings. Then you closed your eyes and paused, noting what you saw or thought in your mind (for the exercise you then wrote down your experiences before turning to the next direction). What was most amazing was the time. What I thought took only ten minutes actually took over three hours.

Whatever your focus, you don't allow the distractions of the world to be present in your mind for this period of time. This is another way of being quiet and at peace (there will be more on this subject in chapter 4).

Prayer

Prayer requires an open and free mind. When you pray, you want your thoughts focused on praise, concerns, or needs. If your thoughts are disturbed by intrusive elements, you will be less able to actually focus on prayer.

Prayer is a marvelous therapy, as are meditation and relaxation. You might feel, by reading this statement, that calling prayer a modality or therapy or remedy is sacrilegious. Prayer is a very special way (and it is a way) to communicate love and healing. Since there are various kinds of prayer, remember that each has special meaning for that time or that person.

Much scientific research has been conducted on the effects of prayer. The people being prayed for in these studies had outcomes of longer life and better healing, even when being prayed for by a person or group located miles away. These effects could not be explained 95 to 99 percent of the time by any other reason.

A group of women prayed for the shrinking of a tumor in the breast of one of their friends. The physician, who did not know about these prayers, was amazed when he examined her that the tumor had shrunk as fast as it did. He decided to remove the tumor sooner than planned, and in checking out the surrounding area found another tumor that had been overlooked and was now as big as the original tumor. These examples go on and on. Some just happened and others were purposefully studied.

Dr. Larry Dossey, M.D., author of *Prayer Is Good Medicine,* has also written *Watch What You Pray For: You Just Might Get It*. He is a physician who set out to prove that prayer had no influential value and researched the subject to the point where he is now its most firm believer. He recognized that bad thought transmitted through prayer, for lack of better words, had as much impact as thoughts with good intentions.

FAITH AND MEDICINE

> "As we enhance our inner capacity for wholeness
> and freedom, we strengthen our outer capacity to love
> and serve."—*Rob Lehman*

Many people with diabetes also suffer from depression. Much of this depression may be induced by blood glucose levels that are too high or too low. Religious attendance predicted lower levels of depression among young Mexican-Americans over three generations. More than a thousand veterans hospitalized for serious problems had half the rate of depression as those who did not find religion to be helpful. In a sample of 451 African-Americans, the more they participated in church services, the less depression was noted for both males and females. Among the 2,956 adults studied, the more a person attended church, the less depression they felt.

Gallup polls have also surveyed faith and medicine. One poll reported that 95 percent of Americans believe in God, and 76 percent reported that prayer is an important part of their daily life. In spite of this recognition, the polls also found that when Americans get sick and most need comfort, spirituality and religion are never addressed as a part of their medical care. (Have you ever asked your health professional to pray with you or for you? You may be hearing more about this as future physicians and up-to-date doctors become more aware of these studies.) There were up to ten three- to five-year awards given to medical schools during 1998 to develop courses about spirituality and medicine to be taught to future physicians. David Larson, M.D., president of the National Institute of Healthcare Research, said, "This points to a new era in medicine—one that focuses on the treatment of the whole person—body, mind, and spirit."

Remember that healing is not necessarily curing. In the field of diabetes, a person might, by using prayer, become more calm. Prayer can lead to more stable blood glucose levels, but the person is not cured of diabetes. We're still looking for scientists to use their God-given gifts to unlock further doors so that a consistently accurate and safe method may be found to cure people of diabetes mellitus.

Allowing yourself to be healed through the use of meditation, prayer, and religious beliefs in a higher power has been confirmed by 75 percent of the more than three hundred studies done on prayer and religious beliefs (reported by Dale Matthews, M.D., associate professor of medicine at Georgetown School of Medicine in Washington, D.C.).

Here are various examples of how religious beliefs, faith, and various practices aid in health:

- African spirituality uses dance to induce a state that refocuses the self and relaxes the mind.
- Catholic priests anoint the sick by putting a drop of oil that has been blessed by a bishop and massaging the oil into the forehead.
- Hindus cleanse their bodies of impurities by fasting or fast on behalf of another.
- Jews visit the sick as one of their commandments and pray for them as part of their religious services.

- Methodists use laying on of hands, anointing the sick with oil, or conduct healing services for those who are ill.
- Mormons have what is called the "Word of Wisdom," a health code written in 1830 that closely resembles today's recommended nutritional guidelines; they also believe in the laying on of hands and administration.
- Muslims have family members read from the Koran to help an ill person be more patient when suffering.
- Native Americans vary in their beliefs from tribe to tribe. A number of tribes use a sweat lodge for healing or to gather to sing and pray.

Herbert Benson, M.D., was able to demonstrate that all religions had some repeated phrase or process that appeared to focus a person's mind away from the trials of the world and thereby result in a state of calmness that more readily allowed healing to occur. More specific studies done by Benson and his staff resulted in a finding that 75 percent of people with sleep disorders were able to obtain quality sleep by using this repetitive process.

To be able to identify the inner peace that is associated with various religious practices and beliefs presented in this chapter, you could weigh the following thoughts adapted from Saskia Davis, printed in the February 1998 issue of *Phase V—The Journey Continues* newsletter of the American Holistic Nurses Association.

Do you have a tendency to think and act spontaneously rather than on fears based on past experience? Do you have an unmistakable ability to enjoy each moment? Have you lost interest in judging yourself and the actions of others? Have you lost the ability to worry? Do you frequently feel overwhelmed by episodes of appreciation for your surroundings and of others? Do you feel connected with others and with nature? Do you find yourself smiling frequently? Do you feel an increased susceptibility to the love extended by others? Do you have an uncontrollable urge to extend love to others?

Each person is just like a recipe. It takes all the ingredients to create the final product. This product is "Wellness and Spiritual Health."*

"Wellness Bouillabaisse Starter Ingredients—genie genes, busy body, smarty smarts, tricky talents, strong strengths, swell cells, can-do fondue;

---

*Wellness Bouillabaisse is adapted with permission from *Diabetes Wellness Letter,* vol. 2, no. 11, 1996. The *Diabetes Wellness Letter* is a publication of the Diabetes Research and Wellness Foundation.

- Physical Health Seasoning Blend Ingredients: fruition nutrition, exercise extract, backward BG, level lipids, faithful meds, sound pounds, deep sleep, smoke free;
- Mental Health Seasoning Blend Ingredients: attitude latitude, nervy nerves, read and seed, thinker toys, trifled trifles, earnest earnest, time outs, R&R;
- Emotional Health Seasoning Blend Ingredients: grandma granules, grandpa garnish, belly laughs, rose snips, back pats, snazzy jazz, together weather, talkie walkie, Friday flakes;
- Spiritual Health Seasoning Blend Ingredients: thoughtful thoughts, heaping hope, fearless faith, integrity inc., fall foliage, Beatles and Bach, grateful heart, holy terriers, helping hands, Psalm 23;
- Social Health Season Blend Ingredients: all-weather friends, parent juice, handy hands, careful causes, chamber chats, tough love, funny fun, evenings out.

Recipe: Use 4 quarts of undistilled water; 1 fistful of Wellness Bouillabaisse starter (do not use Soup Starter); 1 lean fillet of physical health, bones intact; 1 large head of clarified mental health; 1 whopper of first-rate social health; 1 bunch of well-washed emotional health; 1 firm center-cut stalk of spiritual health.

Directions: Trim bruises from the emotional health and carefully inspect mental health for holes that may be hiding large blocks. Discard blocks and bruises. Remove withering leaves from the spiritual stalk and trim the social health so that it fits nicely into the bouillabaisse pot. If you don't have quite enough of one ingredient, it is possible to compensate by adding a little more of the other ingredients, plus large amounts of the seasoning blends. Whisk all ingredients in a large sturdy pot and place on the front burner of the stove. Rapidly bring to a gentle boil, reduce heat, and simmer to blend individual flavors. Stir frequently to keep ingredients suspended in broth. Add seasoning blends according to your own taste, but do add them. Alter this recipe only on advice from gourmet wellness bouillabaisse experts.

If your bouillabaisse doesn't smell or taste quite right, check the following:

1. Check your recipe card for date. If over a year old, consult your advisory chefs for updates.
2. Check the expiration date on seasoning blends. If they are outdated, go shopping.

3. Check the bottom of the pot for ingredients that may have settled. If they're burnt, do not stir. Throw this batch out and start over.

If all fails, develop your own recipe for the balance needed in your life, including an extra check for your environment and for the spirituality in your life."

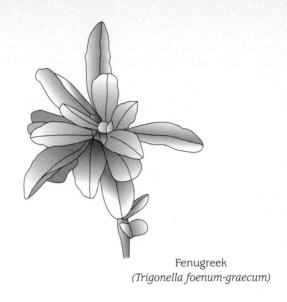

Fenugreek
(Trigonella foenum-graecum)

3

DEALING WITH CONFLICT

Natalie applied for a job. On the application was a place to list illnesses. The only reason she did not list diabetes was that she did not consider herself ill. She met all the qualifications that the position required.

After she was offered the position, her next step was a visit to the company physician. Her blood sugars were usually intensively controlled, but she had a cold and was having to supplement her usual doses of insulin to keep her blood sugars down. The physician saw her laboratory results and stamped her paper as "unemployable" without even seeing her.

She called in tears, telling me what happened. I called the American Diabetes Association's local chapter and reported what had occurred. They recognized that diabetes is often considered a handicap but affirmed that legally no one may be excluded because of diabetes from a job for which they qualify.

The company was in trouble. The vice president of the company was contacted and, after learning about the situation, saw that she was hired.

The results? Over the years, she became the top salesperson in the city, the state, and the region. Later, she came in third in the country.

Thank goodness she was willing to be assertive and call someone and that her local chapter was assertive enough to follow through on an injustice.

ASSERTIVENESS

Assertiveness is often the fine line between what you want to say and what you need to say. Too often, you might feel that it is too difficult to tell someone you have diabetes or make a special food request at a restaurant. At other times you might feel angry and demand that something be done to assist you in your self-care.

Assertiveness was first described by Andrew Slater in 1949, who thought it was a personality trait that some people had. It was later redefined as "expressing personal rights and feelings." Later research found almost anyone could be assertive.

Assertiveness is displaying and using the socially acceptable amount of action and pressure to get what you need to get done without stepping on someone else's toes in the process. Once you have aroused resistance or anger in another person, no matter how subtle, you have become aggressive.

Aggressiveness is expressing your feelings but at the expense of someone else's feelings. You have entered into their field of action. You have used more force and language than is acceptable for the present culture.

Then there are times when you don't want to impose on anyone but you reach a limit where you feel it is about time that your needs be considered. The result is you act out in an angry way. This is termed being passive aggressive and indicates an individual who is not assertive enough to get his or her everyday needs met but when aggravated, goes overboard in expressing those needs.

Self-Efficacy

Self-efficacy is the belief that you can carry out a certain action. This requires having the knowledge and ability to perform that action. This goes along with assertiveness, for if you believe that you are able to do something, you are more apt to make the effort to do it. Since self-efficacy is considered to be the ability to do something, you could do that something assertively or aggressively (stepping on someone's toes). If you are suddenly pushed into doing something in which you are not comfortable, you may not wish to do it. You are told to monitor your blood sugars. You decide you don't want to do it, so you can either yell at the doctor or family member who made the suggestion (aggressive) or you can talk about alternatives about how to do it less painfully (assertive).

If someone suddenly pushes you into an action that you don't like and you get angry and punch a hole in the wall rather than making your concerns known (passive aggressive), then you need to ask yourself if you are willing to determine how this task might most successfully be carried out.

One area of self-efficacy that has been studied says that people with diabetes can recognize when their own blood glucose levels are high or low. Research on this topic revealed that when their blood sugars are too high or too low, individuals who have either Type 1 diabetes or Type 2 diabetes may feel similar symptoms. People do recognize a change of signs or symptoms in their body, but the majority of times they are not able, without adequate training, to determine if the blood glucose levels are elevated or depressed. Being stimulated by the irritability of the too high or too low blood sugar, you might be aggressive and demand a certain treatment, only to find out that your blood glucose levels were the opposite of what you thought they were.

Directly or indirectly, blood glucose levels may influence your assertive responses and turn them into an uncontrolled aggressive response, or if it is your habit not be assertive, turn you into a passive aggressive monster. Therefore, being able to recognize some of the same influences blood glucose levels can have might lead you to recognize that every part of your life has the potential for problem behavior. That is why this chapter includes information on conflict resolution, negotiating skills, forgiving, and coping, plus skills for handling grief, whether in yourself or others.

Conflict Resolution

Conflict resolution, or conflict management, has come of age. It is closely associated with negotiating skills, for one part of this process should not be separated from the other. First, we have to assume that human beings do things for a purpose and, therefore, make choices to meet their needs. Outside stimuli might influence such choices, but people do not necessarily respond just because they feel stimulated to respond. (At work or in relationships, you have probably found that lying is not easy.) It is hard work to keep a good relationship stable. It is a give and take. It is a shared experience.

For example, you may find that your job expectations do not allow time for you to eat your midmorning or midafternoon snack. This puts you in conflict with your supervisor at work. You could get upset about this or you could talk with your supervisor as to how best to work this out. Educating your supervisor about your regimen and about diabetes would be a method to resolve this conflict.

Share this situation with a support group. (If one is not available in your area, go to your local diabetes organization and help them start these monthly "talk time" meetings.)

Communication

Communication is how you share experiences. But you usually communicate only a small part of what you recognize as your ideas or feelings or wishes. Maintaining good relationships involves sharing likes and dislikes, visions or concerns, and hopes and fears. Problems may arise just from how you use your communication skills especially if you are focused more on the past than the present. The past might be represented by a family member who you feel is always nagging you to eat right. The present might be represented by spending some time with that person, sharing concerns about your feelings.

Tools in communication include using the terms "I" and "we" more frequently. The use of the word "you" can lead to defensiveness, such as, "You make me so upset when you tell me I can't eat that because I have diabetes." It comes across more acceptably when the person says, "It concerns me when you try to remind me about what I should eat." The words are softer. They indicate personal feelings rather than accusatory statements. The other person is less apt to be defensive when hearing these words than when hearing the former words. Communicate with others by reflecting feelings, paraphrasing or restating what has been said, and clarifying what you are hearing so there is no doubt what the message means. When you are negotiating with another, you want your words to come across as smoothly as possible and be understood clearly.

Negotiation

> "If one person wins, both lose." —*Author unknown*

Negotiation is truly an art—the art of communicating effectively. It is also an art of compromise. Conflicts may not be resolved unless compromise is addressed. To effectively negotiate requires an ability to give a little or to compromise. Giving this little bit should be done in such a way that you don't feel the worse for it. Communication also involves self-efficacy. As noted before, this is the belief that you can do it; for example, you can communicate effectively or you can identify body signals that tell you when you need to negotiate, as well as having the internal strength to follow through on what you set out to do.

Communication, compromising, and negotiation are tools that assist in changing your behavior for better or worse. Your interpretation, through communication, about what you hear or observe will influence your decision to do or not do something. To succeed in negotiating with your health professional as well as those at work, school, or home also requires the ability to tolerate some discomfort through compromising. All this requires controlling your emotions so that words you use to effect change can be understood intellectually. If you are leading with your emotions rather than listening with your intellect, changes in behavior are not as apt to occur.

Negotiating requires staying in the here and now and determining the importance of both yours and the other person's needs. When you weigh out these needs, determine the pros and cons of whatever you expect as the outcome of your actions. Brainstorm with others to determine if there are alternatives.

For instance, if you read about a new herb in the field of alternative and complementary care that is supposed to cure diabetes, then before you stop taking your medicine, negotiate with your health professional. Learn the possibilities of its use and also the potential problems and share and discuss the information before making a decision or change. Consider what you could do safely.

For instance, if you had Type 2 diabetes, especially if it was well controlled, would there even be any reason to try it? If your Type 2 diabetes was not well controlled, would it hurt to try it for a few days? Learn if this could or could not be a problem.

Then consider your priorities. Is it worth it to try this herb at this time? Have you done enough homework to really know about its actions? Have you been aggressive rather than assertive so that your family or friend or health professional have been put at odds with your reasoning?

Obtain some mutual agreement. Write it down so you and the other person have not misunderstood each other. If a goal or mutual agreement has not been reached within a period of time, be willing to compromise.

This is the win-win format you may have read about. It allows each person involved in the decision-making process to take a side, but in an informed manner. It leaves feelings that are not hurt. It assists in accomplishing what you might wish to happen without making enemies or without compromising safety.

There are many ways to reach this goal. Perhaps your health-care provider has not asked the questions that could lead to the variation in your program that would better meet your needs—or perhaps you have not thought to share what needed to be shared, or you have not completed blood glucose monitoring that would give more guidance to your health professional.

Conflict can arise. You may want to try a particular therapy, but your health professional says it's not good for you because it has not been studied scientifically. You say it has not been studied scientifically but it has been around for over a thousand years. Share what you have read and perhaps talk about doing something on a trial basis.

First, you must demonstrate respect for the other person by giving that person the time to share his or her views. Certainly you both should agree that confidentiality be maintained. You may not want that person to be telling the world that you want to try acupuncture for your neuropathy; neither does that person want it known that he or she doesn't know a thing about acupuncture. Offer and accept another's perspective of the issue without feeling that you have to convince the other person about your views or knowledge. Watch your language! Be sure it does not insult the other person or persons. Rather than "doctor hopping," commit to working it out with that professional so long as that person is able to maintain an open mind.

As you proceed, check whether you are really (really) listening. Note what you think the speaker is feeling. Note whether what he or she is saying restates or reflects what you think has been said or expressed or whether his or her body language reflects what the person is really feeling. For example, you might observe that person tapping a foot in irritation yet saying, "It doesn't bother me." If you're not sure what the person said or if you feel that you have not been heard, repeat what you have said in a different way. Reflect the feelings of the person across from you in as few words as possible, such as, "You're angry because I'm not choosing to do exactly as you told me to." Put a name to your own feelings. Be sure you are understood before continuing.

Share your thoughts on the matter in as respectful a way as possible. Be sure you have studied the matter so that the listener will recognize that you don't want your decision to be a blind one. If you realize that your health professional just does not know enough about a subject, then learn together or call in someone who does know. If they are not sure, give them a copy of an article or a list of materials to read. Come back again at another time to continue the discussion until a compromise or decision can be reached.

Watch out for communication roadblocks. Check yourself to see if you are telling the other person what you are going to do, especially when talking about something controversial like starting megavitamin therapy. Are you threatening by saying you'll go seek help elsewhere? Be careful not to lecture. You may have more knowledge than your practitioner about a certain therapy, but share the information in a positive way. Be careful of negatively criticizing a person directly or indirectly (behind that person's back). Gordon Thomas has written a book entitled *Parent Effectiveness Training*. Read what he says about communication roadblocks.

Check yourself out. Determine how you act in a conflict. How do you relate to the following proverbs? "Might overcomes right." "Tit for tat is fair play." "Getting part of what you want is better than not getting anything at all." And there's that famous one, "He who fights and runs away, lives to fight another day." Reflect if you "Kill your enemies with kindness." Do you stay away from people who disagree with you?

I prefer the following statements made by Sitting Bull: "Let us put our heads together and see what life we will make for our children," and "Gentleness will triumph over anger." Call the American Association of Diabetes Educators (800-338-3633) for the source of a test promoted by Ginger Kanzer-Lewis using these and other proverbs to help you identify how you act in conflict.

Initially, you should focus on the way you negotiate rather than on the conflict itself. Always leave yourself an opening to retreat to and feel accepting of that place. Not all conflicts are won. If a health professional gives you information that reveals that the particular herb you have chosen will not safely leave your body because of the condition of your kidneys, agree not to proceed with using that herb. The purpose of negotiating and resolving a conflict is not to be a winner or a loser but to reach a solution as part of a compromise, a decision, even a collaboration.

There are a number of unfair negotiating skills that some try to use in attempting to resolve a conflict. Do you find yourself attacking the other person's weak areas, for instance, pitting your greater versus their lesser knowledge of a subject? Do you find yourself hassling so that you get your way? Have you found yourself making an unreasonable request and then exploding when you don't get the answer you seek?

Perhaps you've called at an inappropriate time or to prove a point you've said something that is out of context. Or you might be the one who brings up the same issue over and over again. If the focus is more on winning than on negotiating, then you should be aware of the saying at the beginning of this section.

COPING SKILLS

You may have read about a number of coping skills such as forgiving, Thought Field Therapy, negotiation, and conflict resolution. All of these coping skills require you to be able to trust: to trust in the other person or trust in yourself or trust in a higher power. You have to have the major belief that in most instances, others will only do those things to help, not harm, you.

This does not mean blind trust. It means learning to discriminate in whom you place your trust. This has been especially confusing to some who put their trust in a health professional and then find their diabetes management worse rather than better.

Coping also includes having self-esteem or being satisfied with yourself. Assertiveness can be a coping skill. If you do not have enough self-esteem to be assertive, then you will have difficulty in being assertive. So lack of self-esteem can lead to lack of direction or the unwillingness to step out and learn. Self-esteem arises out of successful experiences along with good feedback from others.

Ideas about developing self-esteem may be obtained through reading and listening to self-help tapes. Writing down your best qualities can also be helpful. When writing these down, recognize that you are not perfect nor were you ever meant to be. Perfection is what, you might say, you are working toward.

Be careful that you don't magnify things out of proportion. Having diabetes is one thing, but if it becomes your whole life or if you deny so much that you don't do anything about it, you are in a state of imbalance and thereby put yourself in a potentially ill state.

Coping is any process that assists you in regaining balance. It enables you to move toward healthier action or thinking. Community resources, exercise, and simple skills aid in this process. Relaxation techniques are an important part of this list, and chapter 4 will help direct you develop the coping technique you might find best for you.

Relaxation and exercise promote a balance of the chemicals in the body. When these chemicals are balanced, a person can think more clearly and the body, as a whole, functions better. When these chemicals are out of balance, blood sugars vary to the point where the mind does not function clearly—a situation called cognitive dysfunction. When cognitive dysfunction occurs, blood glucose levels are usually too high or too low. This disturbs your ability to learn and to communicate.

Effective use of leisure time aids in keeping you from dwelling on items that do not promote physical or mental health. For example you could volunteer for a good cause, or support others (such as in a diabetic support group), or be a part of a research study, or learn a new skill, like playing the guitar.

Coping also involves developing healthy relationships. This could be a relationship with yourself or with others. Reading this book will help you to know more about yourself. Finding out about the resources in your community that are available to you also helps you plan how to improve future interactions. As you improve relationships, you also increase your level of trust.

To develop healthy relationships, list your strengths and weaknesses. Think about how your strengths and weaknesses would fit into the development of healthy relationships.

Handling Grief

Negotiating and conflict resolution are, in reality, coping skills as well as assertivness techniques. The way you handle grief is another coping skill. You may feel grief when diagnosed as having diabetes mellitus or having a complication of the disease. These feelings of grief can lead to your becoming obsessed with your loss of good health. You might say to yourself, "I'll never be able to scuba dive again," or "Now they'll never let me play on the team." Losing good health is experienced as being just as serious as the loss of a beloved person or pet. You must address your grief so that life can go on.

You might wish to journal your feelings and thoughts. You might talk to another person about your feelings of grief. Even if medication is prescribed, try to use counseling concurrently with the taking of a medication.

What is most important at this time is to determine if you are participating in healthy bereavement. For instance, you might stop taking insulin because a mate has walked out on you and you figure it was due to your having diabetes. Or, perhaps you stopped medications purposefully because you knew that being hospitalized would give you the attention you were not getting at home.

If you find yourself feeling a genuine sense of hopelessness, if you have withdrawn, or if you find yourself crying uncontrollably, you could be in trouble. Panic attacks or problems with breathing are other red flags that something needs to be done. Getting to the right resource will aid in preventing negative thoughts about using substances that would be harmful to your body, or even thoughts of suicide.

Most cities have a crisis line that you can call. Take time to talk. Allow that person to help you focus on what life means to you. It could be an animal or human that depends on you. There may be a pet or person at work or at home who waits for you. Remember, no one can ever do what you're doing exactly as you do.

If a crisis line is not available, find a person who will listen to your story—by phone or otherwise. Recognize that these are your emotions and accept them at face value. If you feel like crying, cry. Social drugs or other medication cannot do the grief work. Their use only delays the mourning process.

Most of all, take time for yourself. Join a support group. Hearing how others have made it through their times of grieving will give you support in working through your own grief.

Going through the stages of grief does take time (about one year for adjustment to the diagnosis of diabetes, or a change of another bodily function due to a complication of diabetes). Anger (often called depression turned outward) and acute grieving could last for six months or more (the literature shows, for the diagnosis of diabetes, an average adjustment period is six to nine months for children and nine to twelve months for adults). The rebuilding process can take eighteen months or longer if the diagnosis is associated with a child.

Psychologists call the first two months bereavement, but then if the more apparent symptoms persist, they then change their diagnosis to major depression. Society does put its limits or red flags on you, but you as an individual need to feel out your own time in relation to your concerns and comfort level.

The following steps can assist you through the grief process. They can be used in relation to a diagnosis that has the potential to be threatening or to the loss of a loved one.

For diabetes, think about yourself (or the person who has been diagnosed). Remember positive things about the way you or the person was. Note the fearful image you now see in regard to your body or that person's body. Assess the differences and the similarities. Allow this process to help you see who you or that person really is at this time. Remember that previous quote: "You are not your body."

Forgiveness

Part of the grieving process includes the act of forgiveness: forgiving yourself or forgiving others. If your child has diabetes, then you might blame yourself, or you might blame your parents for "giving" you diabetes. In either case, personal forgiveness in needed. Grudges not only keep people apart but also keep you apart from your true self.

If this forgiveness is not given, it can "poison" the soul. This negative thinking can keep you from coping with life and diabetes.

Once you have identified what is to be forgiven and put it in its proper perspective, the annoyances more readily disappear and there is a greater chance that you will forget such incidents. Misplaced pride or a sense of self-importance may keep you from letting go. A person in your life may develop a false position of strength over you when you are feeling such weakness.

Not forgiving could lead to continued agitation and therefore more abnormal blood sugars. Forgiving another is therapeutic, and to forgive yourself or others is to allow personal growth. Sometimes you need to learn to forgive.

Research carried out at the University of Wisconsin–Madison, suggests that once people who are angry or depressed are able to forgive, it improves their emotional health. Since being angry at yourself or others is stressful, and since stressors stimulate the release of counterregulatory hormones (for example, adrenaline, cortisol, etc.), stress results in diabetes management becoming more difficult.

If you look at the big picture of life, sweating the small stuff only makes life more unbearable. Relationships within the family can be molehills that are turned into mountains. When you feel angry, determine if it really is important to you and if taking action or saying something harmful is worth it. Are you sending the right signals?

Thought Field Therapy

"Never lose a chance of saying a kind word."
—William Makepeace Thackeray

Thought Field Therapy (TFT) (or the Callahan Techniques—800-359-2873) is a way to assist you in working through traumatic times. People are especially trained in these techniques as practitioners. Therapy includes the use of treatment points and algorithms, the most famous of which are the patterned tapping of the body as well as the use of eye movements and sound or voice technology. A reported case revealed more therapeutic change occurred in two sessions than over the previous twenty years of psychotherapy.

Another psychologist reported that she had positive responses in 80 to 90 percent of her clients using TFT. These successes were in people with migraines, obsessive compulsive disorders, attention deficit problems, and fibromyalgia.

To date, TFT has not been reported useful in helping those with diabetes—but this might be a technique to consider as a collaborative one with your health professional or with an individual who is trained or willing to obtain the training.

Summary

Remember, you cannot change others, but you surely can change yourself if you work at it. Be sure you are communicating clearly. Be sure what you are saying with your body and facial expression matches what you say in words. Be assertive enough to state your feelings and what you want. Emphasize the best in the other person or in yourself. Learn to "chill out," by using your coping skills such as meditation or journaling.

Ellen Michaud, a writer for *Prevention Magazine,* notes that "it takes five positive encounters a day to cancel out the effects of one negative one. So take the time each day to smile . . . and to hug." Each day, do something to calm yourself and aid, in so doing, in the calming of others.

Finally, look to the long-term consequences related to what you are doing. How healthy are they? Can you choose your foods and test your blood without thinking, "Do I have to do this again?" Are such thoughts or statements going to interfere with your ability to cope? Perhaps you need to focus on how the information or the choice results in your feeling better and allowing you to be more active or assertive.

Determine the role of assertiveness in your life. Then review your coping skills and recognize how they might be used. Determine what you are doing now or how coping skills might complement what you are doing now to get you through the day.

Follow these steps:

1. List your rights, wants, needs, and feelings.
2. Determine the problem associated with these rights, wants, needs, or feelings.
3. Write these problems down.
4. Discuss these problems with the appropriate person or group.
5. Help the person you're talking to understand why what you identified as a problem is important to you, and use the basic *I* words without whining, accusing, or threatening.
6. Reinforce what you wish in a simple, short sentence or two.
7. Make a statement about how both of you will gain. Work toward a "win-win" outcome.

You might use these suggestions during free time at work or with your health professional or other person identified as related to the problem. Consciously use good body and verbal language: eye contact, erect posture, clear speech, no inappropriate laughter, and no unnecessary movements of your arms or legs, including the folding of your arms.

Developing coping techniques, such as being assertive, will allow you to feel in control of your environment rather than sensing that your environment has control of you.

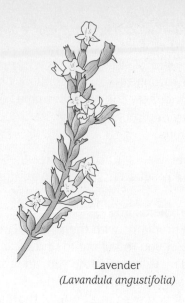

Lavender
(Lavandula angustifolia)

4

RELAXATION: FACT OR FANCY

Tom sat on the edge of his chair as he related what was going on in his life and with his diabetes. He wrung his hands over and over again. He finally mirrored my position in the chair and sat back into his chair. His blood glucose levels were bouncing all over the place. His physician has suggested that he obtain some relaxation training.

His biofeedback-enhanced relaxation training required eleven sessions before he was able to tense and relax at will (the graduation exercise). At each session, he was required to bring in his blood sugar monitoring results. After he was taught diabetes self-management and he became more relaxed, he recognized the need for less insulin (if he did not decrease his insulin doses, he would find himself having hypoglycemic or low blood sugar episodes).

Now he was able to relax at will (in just a few minutes) by "putting his thoughts and deadlines" into a "book," and hearing his quieting music in his mind. If terrifically tense, which he says seldom occurs now, he does a body scan to see which muscles are the most tense and purposefully relaxes them. His blood glucose control has gone from fair to terrific (that is, intensively controlled, with few if any more than mild insulin reactions).

RELAXATION

The ability to relax is something with which you are born. Have you ever observed a sleeping infant? This sleeping infant represents the true state of relaxation. The infant is not disturbed if you raise an arm or leg; its limbs are limp and fall comfortably when released.

What does a relaxed state do for you and how does it fit into your life? The next few pages will contain various ways to practice relaxation.

We need to practice relaxation because we have drifted so far from the true state found in infancy. Learning how to allow ourselves to relax is a process that takes time, but little energy. Why practice?

Have you ever heard anyone say, "I tried to do that relaxation stuff but it just didn't work." People who have *tried* to go to sleep have run into the same difficulty as the person who tried to relax. Trying to go to sleep just causes you to be more wide awake. Trying to relax appears to lead to increased tension rather than a calm and peaceful condition.

PHYSIOLOGY OF STRESS

The relaxed state, physiologically, leads to a slower pulse rate, a slower breathing rate, and a more appropriate use of consumable oxygen. Your nerves are on hold. Adrenaline, associated with the sympathetic nervous system or "flight or fight" response, has its source tucked away in the center (the medulla) of the adrenal gland.

The adrenal glands are somewhat like oranges. There is the inner fruit (the medulla) and the outer skin (the cortex). Most of the secretions of the adrenal gland are associated with adrenaline or cortisol. Adrenaline is secreted from the medulla in response to the sympathetic nervous system (controls the "fight or flight" mechanism). Cortisol is secreted from the cortex in response to the parasympathetic nervous system needs (the day-to-day activities of the body, like thirst, heartbeat, and bowel contraction). When the body is on alert, as in a crisis, adrenaline is released from seconds to minutes, while cortisol's response goes from minutes to hours.

When a sudden alert is sounded in the body, the center part of the brain, or the hypothalamus, sends a message to the middle part of the adrenal gland to release adrenaline. Adrenaline increases the heart rate, increases the blood pressure, and releases stored glucose from the liver and muscle cells into the bloodstream for quick energy.

If this alert is prolonged or intense enough, cortisol or other similar hormones are also released through the message sent from the hypothalamus to the anterior portion of the pituitary gland and on to the outer aspect of the adrenal gland. The release of cortisol elevates the blood pressure, lowers the pulse rate, and changes protein and other sugars into new glucose, ready to be released into the bloodstream.

It is also known that the white cell count decreases in the presence of cortisol. The blood sugar level rises, and a person with diabetes experiencing stress gets an abrupt change in blood glucose levels when, in fact, they may not have eaten a bite of food. Here they have been doing everything they have been told, and in five to fifteen minutes or more, they have documented blood glucose levels starting in the 100s (5 mmol/L +) and rapidly rising to 300s or higher (16 mmol/L +).

Heart attacks or strokes can occur in response to the release of adrenaline. Blood pressure elevation, along with the added pulse pressure and pulse rate, may alter or stress any previously damaged blood vessel walls. If they are too fragile, the blood vessels can break, and a heart attack, or stroke, or hemorrhaging aneurysm occurs.

There is also an association between the presence of cortisol and the lowering of the white blood cell count. Fewer white cells could be the culprit in the increased presence of the *H. pyloris* organism, which is now known to be the cause of stomach ulcer formations.

Adrenaline and cortisol are just two of the many counterregulatory hormones that directly or indirectly influence the level of glucose in the bloodstream. Other such hormones are thyroid stimulating hormone, growth hormone, glucagon, or other hormones from the various glands found in the body. Glucagon is released from the islet of Langerhans' alpha cells that also have cells that release insulin (beta cells).

Insulin is the only counterregulatory hormone that results in the blood sugar going down rather than up. But if a person becomes more agitated and moves about more than usual, the blood sugar could also go down rather than up when he or she becomes stressed. The person is in trouble unless a balance is reachieved between the blood sugar and the brain's need for glucose.

Genetics and Stress

Genes are a very important factor in relation to how the human body will function in the presence of stressors. A stressor can be noise pollution; air pollution; water pollution; problematic family, work, or school matters; and more. Stressors are what cause stress responses, in relation to an individual's genetic makeup.

Change is a stressor. Examples of stressful change are a move to a new location, the start of a new job, a death in the family, a wedding, or a diagnosis of a diabetes complication. Stressors may arise internally—such as thoughts—or externally, such as responses to noise or pollution. The very way you think might make your blood pressure higher. The stress response might result in tight muscles or feelings of anxiousness.

Recognition of the stressors in your life is the first thing to do whenever you are considering a stress management program. Stressor recognition can be of assistance in determining what mechanism you choose in training yourself *to allow yourself* to relax.

Becton Dickinson, a company that produces insulin syringes, has a getting-started pamphlet titled "Diabetes and Stress." It notes that stress can affect your blood sugar, cause your body to make ketones, make you upset, or worse, cause you to stop taking care of yourself. These stress responses can occur abruptly or can become chronic, leading to other diseases or conditions that would interfere with your diabetes condition.

Genes form the basis of the body's response to stressful situations. Further, your genetics are the basis of a model that is useful in determining a stress management program, especially one that may involve alternative or complementary practices. Your genetics will influence the way your body functions when stimulated by an internal or external stressor. The *Diabetes Wellness Letter* referred to the work of Dr. Bruce McEwen and his team from Rockefeller University. They identified stress responses caused by various stressors. As noted previously, the body responds to stressors by increasing blood pressure and decreasing the immune response.

They also found that a stressed person appeared to have an increased deposit of fat around the abdomen, along with weaker muscles, bone loss, increases in blood sugar and cholesterol levels, and increased levels of steroid hormones such as cortisol. A person's genetics monitor how changes in the body take place, and one person may be more sensitive in responding to changes than another.

If you allow yourself to respond to the stressors in your life (for example, a boss who seems to keep picking on you), you could release more adrenaline, which releases more sugar in your bloodstream, which causes you to release (Type 2) more insulin, or need (Type 1) more injectable insulin. In response to this stress you could eat more, but if this "food" can't get into the muscle cells, it will get into the fat cells—with weight gain the probable outcome.

Perceptions

> "Do what you can with what you have, where you are."
> —*Theodore Roosevelt*

How you perceive something is more than 50 percent based on genes rather than experiences. Some experiences will influence perceptions, but in most instances, your differences in perception from your neighbor's will mean that how he or she experiences a frightful situation will be perceived much differently from yours.

This framework then uses three overlapping circles to represent the mental (or intellectual functioning), the physical, and the emotional functioning of the body. Where these circles overlap, you might call the spiritual (ideas, religious beliefs, health beliefs, self-worth, self-esteem, etc.). The larger the overlap, the more balanced the person's life and the more spiritual that person has become.

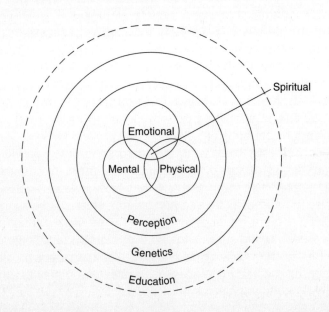

EDUCATION (THE MOST IMPORTANT THING)

The thread that interlinks the spiritual, the mental, the emotional, the physical, the perceptual, and the genetic is education. Through education we can understand how all these parts function and interrelate. It allows the impossible to happen. A person using rapid-acting insulin (insulin administered right before meals) may find that awkward schedules that could not be tolerated before can now be handled effectively and safely (for example: a person who changes shifts from days to nights, to evening, etc., throughout the week or month).

Education plays a role in improving self-esteem, and it might be looked at as the connecting link or thread. This is not to say that the spiritual is less important, but in this day and age, education may be required to assist people in recognizing the spiritual qualities in their lives and how they and the other interrelated parts affect their diabetes. In turn, education helps the person with diabetes to recognize what he or she can accomplish in spite of having diabetes.

RELAXATION AND THE MANAGEMENT OF DIABETES

Research has demonstrated how relaxation lowers and stabilizes blood glucose levels. It is possible for a person trained to relax on self-command to have the capability of lowering blood glucose levels in a matter of twenty to thirty minutes. The major concern was that when the relaxation practice occurred before a meal or snack, or at a time when the full impact of the medication was happening, there would be a greater chance of hypoglycemia. But if practice sessions are held after a meal or snack then this is not a problem. The outcome is that relaxation practice does appear to stabilize as well as lower blood glucose levels.

Appropriate medical management, such as lowering the hypoglycemic medication prior to the time blood sugars are lower, prevents hypoglycemia from being a problem. Rapid swings in the blood glucose levels are less frequently documented when the person develops a more calm and controlled manner by being able to relax at will. Training for relaxation may be enhanced and speeded up by the use of biofeedback.

Biofeedback

Biofeedback is a process involving the use of certain mechanisms, such as temperature, heart rate, blood pressure, electromyography (electricity released by muscles [EMG] much like the electricity released and documented in obtaining an electrocardiogram [ECG], electroencephalogram

[EEG]), blood glucose monitoring, etc. Biofeedback information could be obtained by observing a "stress ring" (a ring center affected by warmth), or pressing a designated area on the "stress card" (a section of a card affected by body heat). Biofeedback could involve the placement of a "stress dot" on the hand (which changes color as your body becomes more relaxed). More sophisticated biofeedback involves the use of sensors and a monitor that are able to tell you your heart rate, blood pressure, temperature, muscle electricity, (EMG), or brain electricity (EEG).

A biofeedback program—whether you could do yourself or with a certified biofeedback therapist (check your phone book or contact a state or national biofeedback association)—may require from seven to twelve weeks for adults to "relearn" the ability to relax. For children, the ability to relax can be retrained in four to six weeks or less. Weekly sessions of feedback reinforcement (along with daily practice sessions at home, using an instrument of some sort such as a handheld alcohol thermometer) can aid you in identifying whether you are relaxed or not. If the temperature rises while you are holding the bulb of an alcohol thermometer, then it indicates that you are more relaxed. A lowering of the EMG or the blood pressure or the heart rate also indicates that you are relaxed.

Early work in the 1970s had people believing that if you had diabetes, especially the insulin-dependent kind, you could not participate in biofeedback-enhanced relaxation training. This advice was based on having feedback and relaxation practice mid- to late afternoon when the subjects were on one dose of NPH insulin (right at the height of the action of the NPH insulin). These people experienced insulin reactions. The concept of reducing and redistributing the insulin didn't appear to be part of their management regimen. The blame was just put on the modality—biofeedback-enhanced relaxation.

My early work demonstrated that if you had a good distribution of insulin and food and practiced biofeedback after a meal or snack, then by carefully monitoring your blood glucose levels and reducing the previous dose of medication when the blood sugars lowered to the 60s or less, hypoglycemia was not a problem. This study concluded that the use of biofeedback with a regulated program was safe for people with diabetes.

This conclusion was replicated through a study completed by McGrady and group. In their work in the late 1980s, they demonstrated that people with elevated blood glucose levels would achieve lower blood glucose levels through the intervention of biofeedback-enhanced (or speeded-up) relaxation training. Relaxation training is now considered a useful intervention in many situations involving highly stressed people with diabetes.

Biofeedback Programs

There are a variety of programs using biofeedback-enhanced relaxation methods. The program I use starts by taking a baseline reading of temperature and EMG during the first session along with a total health assessment (how you are eating, sleeping, exercising, working, believing, and general health). The baseline is useful to compare a participant's later response to training. The patient is also asked to complete a Myers-Briggs Personality Inventory and to choose a tape to be used during their relaxation practice time (preferably two times a day). Tapes from which to choose might include progressive relaxation, or autogenic therapy, or deep breathing, or music of interest, or self-help information, or someone using metaphors or stories. Whatever the tape chosen, the purpose is to keep your mind focused on something so that it is not disturbed by the problems of the day.

The purpose of the second week's session is to see whether the tape chosen has a positive rather than a negative effect on relaxation ability. This positive effect is determined by the temperature going up and/or EMG going down. When the third week arises, the person is able to view the monitor screen to see how the body's muscle electricity (EMG) and temperature respond to various stimuli. By the fourth or fifth week, the pre- and post-temperature notations and the continuing journaling of responses start to form a pattern that leads to the discovery of a cue. A cue is a word, thought, poem, scripture, prayer, or visualization that focuses the attention of the person with an association to relaxing. From then on, each time the person practices (still preferably twice a day), he or she first thinks about the cue, which reminds the body that it is time to become quiet and loose.

Part of sessions six and seven can be used for independent practice while hooked up to the machines. This is to allow the individual to become more aware of his/her own responses without feeling as if someone is peering over his/her shoulder.

The eighth and ninth visits are the times when reports are given about the practices or use occurring outside the home, along with the more sophisticated responses elicited by the machines. If by session ten, or before, the person is able to tense and relax at will, the individual "graduates."

Use of Biofeedback

Biofeedback, as noted before, is useful for changing various behavior patterns. One good example is the treatment for bruxism (teeth grinding). With the use of EMG, which makes a grinding noise when you grit your teeth, a person can stop this habit within a few days or weeks.

Biofeedback also aids people with diabetes to relax and open up blood vessels in hands and feet. If you have a problem with migraines, biofeedback can aid in decreasing the frequency and intensity of these episodes not caused by anything other than tension. It aids in lowering blood pressure, slowing heart rate, and controlling tics or other annoying habits.

Scientific studies have shown that the relaxation response alone has been effective in altering hypertension, cardiac arrhythmias, chronic pain, insomnia, side effects of cancer therapy, side effects of AIDS therapy, anxiety, hostility, depression, premenstrual syndrome, infertility, and preparation for surgery or X-ray procedures.

Breathing Practices

"For fast-acting relief, try slowing down." —*Lily Tomlin*

Deep breathing aids in relaxation and especially in eliciting the relaxation response. The "relaxation response" was studied and reported by Dr. Herbert Benson, a noted physician and professor at Harvard Medical School (see page 30). He observed that anxious people breath shallowly—usually termed "chest breathing." This may sound familiar, but deep breathing has been shown, as was also noted by Dr. Andrew Weil in his newsletter, *Self Healing* (800-523-3296), to lower blood pressure, decrease or stop heart arrhythmias, improve digestion, increase blood circulation, decrease anxiety, and improve sleep quality.

Deep breathing also aids in stress reduction. To practice this, lie on a flat surface with a book placed on your abdomen. As you breathe in (inhale), observe the book go up. As you exhale or breathe out, see the book lower. Then use this technique when you need to calm yourself.

Breathing can also be used to enhance the learning process. A Romanian breathing technique uses background baroque music as a relaxing way to learn more effectively. The beat of certain baroque music corresponds to the rate of a heart beating. One procedure involves breathing in, to the count of two, holding your breath to the count of four while reading your material, and then breathing out for two counts (the counts corresponding with the beat of the music).

It is also possible to enhance your test-taking practices by taking two or three deep breaths at the beginning of a test. You should then answer the questions that easily come to mind. The second time through the test, breathe deeply a few times before trying to answer the questions you know that you have studied but whose answers you couldn't remember the first time through. The third time through, on multiple-choice questions, rule out the obvious incorrect answers and then guess. You have a 50 percent chance of being right. Using this type of breathing has been shown a number of times to result in higher grades.

Another method of relaxing breathing is what Dr. Weil describes as the yoga-style breathing. You start by sitting with your back straight or lying in a comfortable position. Place the tip of your tongue to the ridge in back of your upper front teeth and keep it there during the entire exercise. Exhale through the mouth with a whoosh sound. Close your mouth and inhale through your nose to the count of four. Hold your breath for seven counts and then exhale, with the whoosh sound, to the count of eight. Do this for four cycles.

One more method of breathing that is popularly used is alternative breathing. After being seated in a comfortable position, close your right nostril with your index finger. Inhale slowly through your left nostril. Release your finger and use the same finger to close your left nostril. Inhale through the right nostril. Start this by doing five cycles. Eventually work up to twenty-five cycles. Be sure to breathe normally for a few minutes before standing.

The Relaxation Response

The relaxation response (the decrease of blood pressure and pulse rate, and the improved utilization of oxygen) revolves around some things you can do and think. To obtain or elicit the relaxation response, you need to focus (perhaps by using deep breathing, or walking), repeat the word *one,* or use other repetitious words, phrases, or mantras (such as the rosary, or "God is love," etc.), and to passively handle outside or intrusive thoughts.

Eliciting the relaxation response has been shown to assist patients with chronic pain and especially pain resulting from fear or loss of hope. Dr. Dennis deLeon, in his article "The Relaxation Response in the Treatment of Chronic Pain" in the *Alternative Medicine Alert: A Clinician's Guide to Alternative Therapies* (1998), found this process most helpful. Although this remedy has not been used specifically with the diabetes population, it has been found to be of help to cancer patients, postoperative patients, and women with severe premenstrual cramps.

The following simple two-step procedure, practiced ten to twenty minutes once or twice a day, can result in the relaxation response:

1. Repeat a word, sound, prayer, phrase, or muscular activity (such as deep breathing) that fits with your belief system.
2. Disregard or ignore everyday thoughts that come to mind, adopt a passive attitude, and continue with no. 1.

To stay on track, you should gently refocus outside thoughts back to the repeated word or phrases, or just try to keep the repeated focus on deep breathing or the type of breathing you choose (in through the nose and out through the mouth).

For all types of relaxation practice—in particular progressive relaxation, autogenic training, Zen, yoga, the presuggestion phase of hypnosis, transcendental meditation, and other simple techniques—the results of the body's relaxation response are: the pulse rate slows, breathing becomes more effective and oxygen is used more efficiently, breathing rate decreases, and blood pressure lowers (not significantly documented in autogenic training and transcendental meditation). Brain waves slow in transcendental meditation and in the use of other simple techniques such as Benson's relaxation response method, but increase in autogenic training, Zen, and yoga.

To obtain the best therapeutic effect, it is better to participate in several short sessions a day (two or more, fifteen minutes plus or minus in duration) than fewer sessions of longer duration.

OTHER WAYS TO RELAX

"White Noise"

Sounds may be used as "white noise," or a focus for relaxation. The sounds of soothing music, waterfalls, ocean waves, birds, or breezes may also be useful. Some teenagers state that hearing classical music is stressful to them, while rock music is stressful to some adults. Most classical music, especially Bach, will have a heart-rate type of rhythm. Interestingly enough, so does rock.

Hard rock, on the other hand, has a counterheartbeat rhythm, so it doesn't directly lead to relaxation. It is possible that such music might "drown out" negative or painful thoughts and by that interference, allow the listener to become more relaxed.

Discordant music has been shown to cause cells, visualized by high powered microscopes, to shrivel, while pleasant music sustains or enhances the cells' shape. Modern music might use discordant notes to create a feeling that is not meant to be relaxing.

Careful choice of music (especially fifty beats per minute) or sound can enhance the relaxation session or become the focus of a session, used alone or along with imagery.

Prayer

Prayer can be specifically about healing or be a healing power itself. "Healthy spirituality is based on a healthy psychology," noted Reverend Joseph J. Driscoll in his talk on Catholic Spiritual Healing Practices for the Harvard Medical School conference Spirituality and Healing Medicine in Dallas, Texas (1998). Prayer to benefit another, or intercessory prayer, has had documented influences on healing—or as Driscoll described healing, "as the process of touching, soothing, and alleviating the disease in the spirit, mind and body of a person or a community."

Virginia S. Harris, in her presentation on Christian Science Spiritual Healing Practices at this same conference, said, "Prayer is the humble recognition of the spirit of the man within."

There is a story about a person who asked Thoreau (who wrote about Walden Pond), "Have you made your peace with God?" His response was, "I didn't know that we had quarreled."

Some prayers can be intense and, therefore, not relaxing. But prayers that include support words and peaceful intentions, especially if they are repetitive prayers, physiologically elicit the relaxation response. Since prayer is so powerful, Larry Dossey, M.D., reminds us to be careful what we pray for as we just might get it. So using prayer for relaxation must be carefully thought out, and the choice of the type of prayer should be carefully considered.

Meditation

Meditation is also useful for relaxation. Meditation has the potential of increasing brain wave output, but it can just as easily decrease brain wave output, depending on the process used; for example, mindfulness meditation, a nonjudgmental awareness of bodily sensations and any mental activity happening at that time, is a program requiring eight weeks of training. Single focused meditation, such as that found in beta/theta training, needs about thirty to forty sessions of training time. Beta/theta training with the use of the electroencephalogram (EEG) has proven useful for aiding both children and adults with attention deficit and addictive problems. Both of these techniques elicit the relaxation response.

Concentrated meditation trains you to passively observe a bodily process (such as breathing), a word, or a stimulus. The famous example is "contemplating your belly button," or gazing at a beautiful picture or view from a window.

Transcendental meditation focuses on a sound or thought (a mantra). It sounds difficult to do, but basically, for example, you focus on a sound (again, the word *one* is useful or "Ohm," as a mantra that stands for wholeness or oneness) without thinking about what the sound means.

Both prayer and meditation can get you in the state Dr. Benson describes as "remembered wellness." This might be compared to the previous example of allowing the body to be in the state found in a sleeping baby.

Visualization

Visualization could be guided (most people refer to this as guided imagery). It could be programmed, such as practicing a golf swing or throwing a basketball. Receptive visualization allows your mind to flow freely with or without a focus (such as a problem) while preparing your body to be relaxed and preparing your mind to be as "empty" as possible ("be" in your special place or reach your "inner guide" or choose a certain color). When you are focusing on that peaceful scene you are visualizing.

Guided Imagery

Guided imagery is a method often accompanied by quieting music or outdoor sounds. It may follow a story or a metaphor (a story that has meaning to you) or mentally guide you to walk down a path in an area that promotes peace and quiet. Compared to relaxation therapy and hypnosis, guided imagery is oriented mentally to the imagination rather than the muscles. While relaxation training is known to alter physiological processes, guided imagery and hypnosis usually elicit such processes, as noted earlier. Interestingly, relaxation therapy may stimulate imagery, and most such guided imagery, depending on the way it is used, appears to result in relaxation.

Self-Hypnosis

Self-hypnosis is also useful for relieving stress. In fact, any therapy that maintains your attention is a form of self-hypnosis. When you are in complete control you can stop doing or thinking whatever you're focused on at any time.

Start by lying or sitting comfortably. Breathe deeply and evenly. Visualize a staircase, elevator, or escalator that moves up or down in relation to your perception of being more relaxed. Each floor or each step allows you to sink deeper into a state of relaxation.

Experience the drowsiness that can occur as you become even more relaxed. You can drift up or down to your special place from which, in this most relaxed state, you may choose to just relax or to find an answer to a problem. Give yourself a "posthypnotic suggestion" such as, on "awakening," I will clearly remember all my thoughts and write them down without any problem.

As you choose to end your session, do the opposite of what you did to become more relaxed, that is, go up or down the stairs, or on the escalator, or elevator, becoming more alert the closer you get to the place you started. Give yourself time to breathe evenly and normally before continuing with your activities. If this method interests you, make your own self-induction tape or check your bookstore for useful resources.

Progressive Relaxation

Progressive relaxation is another method. Dr. Edmund Jacobson, developer of this method, noted in 1938 that people often don't know how to relax a muscle because they don't know how a relaxed muscle feels. One of the major purposes of progressively contracting and relaxing muscle groups is to determine how these muscles feel tense, so that you can know how the muscle feels in the relaxed state.

With this method, you usually start with the muscle groups of the toes. You curl them or tense them in the way you suppose muscles feel when tight. Hold them in that position for a number of seconds and then relax or loosen those muscles, observing how they feel once the muscles are relaxed.

You would next progress to the feet, then the muscles of the ankles, the calves of the legs, and so forth. You would proceed all the way to the top of the head, including all body parts. The last tensing of muscle groups would be the "scrunching up" of the face and subsequently relaxing that area of the body.

Practicing this process for a period of time would eventually get you to the state where you could progressively focus on that part of the body and sequentially sense, from one muscle group to another, whether the muscle fibers are truly in a relaxed state or not.

You would be able to do this without even having to first contract the muscles. But to strengthen this process of relaxation, maintain the practice of contracting and relaxing to allow the muscle fibers to "learn" to relax even more.

Autogenic Therapy

Johannes H. Schultz is responsible for developing autogenic therapy (Wolgang Luthe is responsible for reporting the research in 1969). This methodology has been used in a wide variety of practices. Originally, it was divided into six standard exercises using specific words. First you focus on the generalized sensation of experiencing the heaviness in your body, arms, and legs. Then you make statements saying you have a feeling of warmth or coolness in your hands, feet, arms, legs, and body. To achieve a normal heart rate you say, "My heartbeat is calm." You can regulate breathing by saying, "It breathes me." To relax and warm the abdominal region say, "My solar plexus is warm." Finally, focus on the reduction of the flow of blood to the head by saying, "My forehead is cool." Each of these standard exercises might individually be used for the duration of two to three weeks before proceeding to do or add the next exercise.

One variation is to use the sequence of muscle groups, as in progressive relaxation, and allowing those muscles to feel heavier and heavier. As those particular areas of the body feel heavier, the physiological response is a more relaxed muscle. When the muscles are more relaxed, there is less pressure on the blood vessels, thereby allowing the blood to flow to the extremities. This results in the sensation of warmth.

If you like an organized method (externally locused), of doing something in a sequence, then you would find progressive relaxation helpful. If you are more laid back, internally locused, and like to use thought as a process for relaxation, autogenic therapy might be your choice.

Aromatherapy

Aromatherapy might be another way to help you sleep relaxed or as an aid in healing. Pleasant aromas will aid you in relaxing (aromatherapy will also be discussed in chapter 7 and in chapter 8.). For relaxation, particular scents can be placed in a room or on the body in a massage oil. The aromas may be stimulating or calming to enhance the body's ability to feel peaceful.

When used as a room scent, you would put aromas in a container of basic oil, such as almond oil, or into a specific container that is heated and, in the process of heating, releases the oil's aroma.

Oils have been used in this way for many, many years, often to cover the smells of the city, or in the past as burnt offerings, or to cover body odor when it was not thought wise to bathe. People experiencing these fragrances were found to be more relaxed than if they smelled odors that were uncomfortable to them.

Sleep

Besides lowering and stabilizing blood glucose levels, relaxation is a way to enhance or improve the quality and quantity of sleep. General recommendations for relaxation and sleep include being sure the temperature of the room is comfortable. Studies show that a room temperature of sixty to sixty-five degrees Fahrenheit is conducive to sleep (but this does conflict with the environmentalists who recognize the energy it takes to keep the temperature that low in the hot days of summer).

It is important to awaken at the same time each morning. Sleeping late, unless there is some real need, actually disturbs the sleep cycle. Ideally, drinks that include caffeine or alcohol should be avoided, limited, or drunk early in the day. Forget the cigarettes and cigars. Remember, exercise is a stimulant. If you don't want exercise to bother your sleep, some say you should exercise no closer than five to six hours before going to bed.

A warm bath (a hot bath or shower also acts as a stimulant), a light snack, and a method of relaxation (e.g., music, imagery, or relaxation technique) should be scheduled each evening as part of the sequence of getting ready to go to sleep. A bedtime snack is useful for most individuals whether they have diabetes or not. It actually helps the human body not get too hypoglycemic during the night and "push" the person into REM (rapid eye movement) sleep before "desired." Also, plan to find out if any of the medications you are taking will bother your sleep. Remember to "allow" yourself, rather than "try," to go to sleep.

Some people only need four to five hours of sleep at night while others need nine to ten hours or so of sleep. Experiment and find out the average number of hours of sleep that allow you to feel most rested. This needs to be done when your blood glucose levels are controlled, for waking up at night numerous times to go to the bathroom or to take an extra snack because your blood sugars are too low does not lead to restful sleep.

Check out your pillow and mattress. Whatever pillow you choose, be sure it gives you enough support for your neck. Air mattresses are popular. They are the same size and shape as the standard mattress with inside chambers that hold air and aid in evenly distributing your weight. Pocketed water beds or the use of a medium-to-firm mattresses with adequate padding are also helpful. Others have found that "magnetic" beds have brought them a better quality of sleep (eight-hour limit recommended). If you ever sleep in a bed that is more comfortable than your own, don't miss the opportunity to find out what kind of mattress is on the bed.

Again, what you sleep on adds to the list of considerations that can help you have the most restful sleep possible. When you sleep well, you can handle about anything. When you feel irritable because of lack of sleep, you are not fit to live with—even though your blood glucose levels might be perfectly normal.

Surprisingly, if all the above does not work, you could use "paradoxical intent." This is a process in which you instruct yourself not to fall asleep. As you try to stay awake you will find yourself getting sleepier and sleepier.

SUMMARY

"To relax is the process of learning how to get out of
your own way so that your body will automatically relax."
—*Diana Guthrie*

Purposeful relaxation assists you in altering your stress responses by addressing your environment, handling social stressors (e.g., deadlines and disagreements), being able to "turn off your brain" or control your thoughts, and recognizing the physical responses of diabetes and life in general and its impact on your body.

Stress responses are not all bad. These responses are useful in preparing you to fight or flee. Without stress responses of some sort, you would not be alive, but though there are beneficial aspects to stress responses, you are all too familiar with the "bad" ones.

You need to assess whether you are a victim of acute or chronic stress and what you have tried that has worked and what has not worked. Become aware of how your body functions. Scan your body for tense areas or injuries. Write down a list of the external stimuli that are a part of everyday life.

If you grew up in a large city, such as New York City, a return visit requires about two days to lose the awareness of the garbage trucks making their 4 A.M. rounds. If you grew up in the country and you are visiting the city, it will take much longer before your brain decreases the awareness of the trucks and their noise.

Some stimuli you can just ignore—they become a part of your environment. Others put you on alert, such as getting up when the alarm clock rings. Journal such things as meetings and paperwork. Note how your body responds to each of these (e.g., a usual night's sleep; a tension headache).

Prevention of tension is best. Think about how you adjust to change.

If you pace yourself and do as much preplanning as possible, you will find you are able to adjust to almost any situation. As you reach a goal, don't consider it a time to stop but acknowledge it as just part of a continuum on your path of life. When you "let down," it is much harder to get your engine going again. This can lead to a life that has more ups and downs than a roller coaster. Once or twice a day, allow yourself the time it takes to become relaxed. With training, look forward to accomplishing this task in just a few minutes. Take these quiet times shortly after you've eaten and use the effect that carbohydrates can have on your body.

There are a variety of catalogs that list resources to be used with self-training. The not-for-profit Conscious Living Foundation (800-578-7377) has tapes for guided imagery and other means to assist you in developing a relaxed state. They also have instrumentation useful for children and adults, such as thermometers that read in one-tenth of a degree. One tape, usually used by children, but helpful for adults, too, has you mentally shrink to a size in which you can get into a blood vessel and travel throughout the body, observing and fixing whatever is "broken." Other tapes describe various scenes and pleasant surroundings and accompany the descriptions with music or natural sounds. Department stores and music stores also carry a variety of cassettes or CDs that contain sounds of nature or types of music pleasing to almost everyone.

Being able to relax when you want to is a challenge and also a skill. You can only imagine what is possible once this skill is mastered.

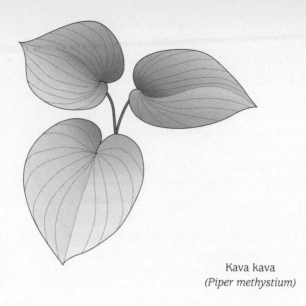

Kava kava
(Piper methystium)

5

PAIN OR PLEASURE

"The way I see it, if you want the rainbow you gotta be willing to put up with the rain." —*Dolly Parton*

Ann reported to her physician the chest pains that she had felt while driving to other side of town where she was to moderate a lecture. Cardiovascular enzymes (blood work) were taken and an electrocardiogram was obtained. All were normal.

When I saw her, she was still having the chest pains, but the physician felt some kind of noninvasive therapy would be of use to her. When she described her lifestyle, the major lack was exercise. She was actually doing other things to de-stress her life, but exercise was not one of them. She felt that exercise in the morning was not an option because of her home responsibilities. After she returned from work, exercise was not an option because she felt too exhausted.

After assessing what she might agree to try, she decided on swimming. The goal the first week was to swim only one lap of the pool.

"The first few days were terrible," she reported, "and then something happened. As I completed the one lap and then started increasing the number of laps by adding a lap every day or so, I found myself feeling better than I ever had."

Not surprisingly, the chest pains were no longer mentioned unless I questioned her directly. They had gone. The endorphins and enkephalins she was producing and releasing into her bloodstream left her with a sense of well-being, a decreased feeling of depression, and "no pain." She is now completing daily, or every other day, about twenty-five to thirty laps. (Blood sugars?—better than they have ever been.)

EXERCISE

Exercise is a subject that some love to talk about and others would rather not. There's a Garfield cartoon in which Jon says to Garfield as he is lying comfortably in his box, "Let's go jogging." Garfield replies, "No thanks, sweatsock breath. Exercise gives me the dry heaves."

This is often the present-day philosophy. But there is so much more to exercising than just the "No pain! No gain" image that the word *exercise* itself gives to most people. You now have a greater choice, from the more intense aerobic types of exercise to the types that are centuries old, such as Tai chi and yoga. Exercise may be aerobic (a greater increase of oxygen use) or anerobic (lesser increase of oxygen use). Increased activity also increases oxygen use. So walk, climb stairs, or stretch a rubber band. Among its other benefits, anything that increases oxygen use also increases endorphins.

Exercise is also the cornerstone of pain prevention. Stretching tones the back and other supporting muscles. Strength training decreases your risk for falls, and, if osteoporosis is present, helps prevent compression fractures.

Regular exercise, performed every day or every other day at about the same time, was identified as one of the cornerstones of diabetes management as early as the 1920s. During the ensuing years, use of exercise has evolved as a science. Because each person is different, each exercise program may be different. Also note that regular exercise may be a protector against age-related mental decline in humans caused by impaired blood flow to the brain.

Whether you have Type 1 or Type 2 diabetes, consideration need to be given for the distribution of food and/or medication during an exercise program. Any person starting on an exercise program is requested to determine the physical capabilities of his or her body. Your physician may have you take a stress test (walk for so long on a treadmill while your breathing and heart rate are recorded), especially if you are older than thirty-five to forty years of age, or older than twenty-one and have had diabetes for ten years or longer. Your eyes should be checked for any signs of blood vessel damage perhaps more often than the recommended yearly check. A good source for in-depth information is a book on exercise that is available through the American Diabetes Association (800-232-3472).

STARTING A PROGRAM

> "I am not discouraged, because every wrong attempt
> discarded is another step forward." —*Thomas Edison*

Before starting a serious exercise program, get that health checkup and an okay from your doctor. Then, start by increasing your level of activity. Take the steps rather than the elevator and park farther away from your destination. Short walks (like ten minutes a day) could be next. Try some different exercises or request to try out some exercise machines at a local health club. Start participating in one or more ways of exercising to help make it more interesting for you.

If you have a VCR, get some aerobic, low-impact aerobic, Tai chi, Qigong, or yoga tapes (call 800-433-6769 for a catalog of exercise tapes), or the more recently popular Tae-Bo (800-637-6632). You could also try out the programs on a fitness channel. For a fee, you could hire a personal fitness trainer to guide you in developing your own program.

Meditation combines well with exercise, as it aids in improving health even more. When walking, swing your arms to aid your legs in providing a better workout. Focus on your breathing or the swinging of your arms. The same should be done with bicycling, jogging, running, swimming, or jumping rope. Paced, rhythmic, flowing movements can bring about a relaxed state while you are working out.

You should include FITT in your program: *Frequency* (usually no less than three times a week at twenty to thirty minutes at each time); *Intensity* (if you are unable to sing or talk while exercising, then you are exercising too hard); *Time* (early morning results in a more than 50 percent chance that you will be exercising a year from now, noon, about a 50 percent chance, and evening, less than a 50 percent chance you'll still be exercising a year from now); and the *Type* of exercise.

It has been demonstrated that exercise can be used to treat mild depression. It also aids in stabilizing blood glucose levels if done regularly.

Heart rate should be checked before, during, and after the aerobic exercise period. (To determine your heart rate, take 220 less your age multiplied by 60 percent and 80 percent to determine the range of heartbeats per minutes.) The older you are, the slower you should start, gradually increasing in time and intensity.

Physiologically, exercise increases and tones heart rate and pulse rate, promotes physical fitness, aids in rehabilitation, decreases depression, increases a sense of well-being, lowers bone mineral loss, relieves back pain, assists in weight control, and supports cardiovascular strength. As you become more conditioned your pulse rate will lower.

When you start exercising, the fuel you use is glucose, which is obtained from glycogen stores and triglycerides (excess glucose is stored in this form of fat in the fat cells). As you continue exercising, you use up the glycogen stores and revert to using fat stores. In the presence of any stressor, and, yes, exercise is a stressor, the body releases free fatty acids. These are used with increasing frequency while exercising. To really use the fats in your body as an energy source (as in weight-loss programs), you need to exercise at least forty-five to sixty minutes. This means that people who have tried and "failed" at exercising should just learn from Thomas Edison and "try, try again." Edison said there were two thousand learning experiences (not failures) before the light bulb was invented. Hopefully, it doesn't take you two thousand trials before you start exercising.

Types of Exercise

There are various types of exercise. The most common types are aerobic, anaerobic, and isokinetic. Aerobic exercises are the most widely used in this country. Oriental countries, especially the older population, use Tai chi (developed to strengthen the military) or Qigong (a form of Tai chi developed by physicians for its healing potential). Tai chi and Qigong involve a series of positions performed in sequence on a daily basis. In India and elsewhere, yoga is the activity of choice. There are eight or more types of yoga, some accompanied by various forms of meditation.

Increased beneficial activity can be obtained from golf, swimming, skiing, other sports, and anaerobic exercise, which is a less intense exercise.

Isokinetic exercise includes strength training, which involves working against a resistance (such as using weight machines or other workout equipment).

A person who has developed retinopathy is cautioned against participating in isokinetic exercises. Isokinetic exercises are those in which the muscles change in length.

Simple walking is one of the most recommended exercises for anybody. One Finnish study that included 16,000 twins for nineteen years found that participants who walked briskly for thirty minutes six times a month or more were 44 percent less likely to have died earlier than their sedentary twin.

Other studies support that walking can boost energy, lower blood pressure, and raise high-density lipoproteins (HDL)—the good fat (cholesterol coming out of the tissues and going back to the liver to be broken down chemically to be eliminated from the body), and reduce the risk of osteoporosis.

Dr. Andrew Weil recommends a walking program that has nine steps:

1. Wear supportive shoes with double-layered socks.
2. Start out slowly, beginning with a few minutes (he says ten) each day until you reach forty-five minutes a day, five days a week.
3. Keep good posture by standing up straight and relaxing your shoulders, and look straight ahead.
4. Swing your arms with each stride, bending your elbows when you wish to increase your pace.
5. Walk on varied inclines by including some hills on your route.
6. Pick up the pace until you are able to walk 140 steps a minute, to equal four miles an hour.
7. Walk with a friend as a motivator.
8. Use music and keep time to the music as you walk (marching music is great for slower walking).
9. Walk whenever you can by parking farther away from the door.

A simple exercise program was given in "Medical Essay," a part of the *Mayo Clinic Health Letter.* The first step is to lie on your back, bending your knees up so that you do a half sit-up. This could be done with both knees together or alternately with each knee-to-shoulder action.

Next, on your hands and knees, let your abdomen sag toward the floor and then slowly arch your back like a cat as comfortably as can be tolerated. Then lie flat on your abdomen with a pillow under your hips and lower abdomen, first bend each leg at the knee and then fully raise the straight leg, holding each position for five seconds. Next, proceed to sit on a chair and slowly bend forward toward the floor until you feel a stretching sensation in your back. Hold for fifteen to thirty seconds. Finally, sit squarely on the chair and squeeze your shoulder blades together a few seconds each time.

Similar exercise programs are stimulating and motivating. There is a growing movement to treat chronic illnesses with exercise rather than with the old approach of conserving energy. If you ever go to the Mayo Clinic, you will notice a stationary bicycle in the rooms of heart transplant patients. These are used by patients only two days after surgery.

Many hospitals host full-size gyms. Although exercise can't cure diabetes or heart disease, it may halt the disease, or it can delay the need for drugs and reverse the toll of high blood sugars and weakened heart muscle and thereby lengthen and improve the quality of life.

Recent documentation that exercise raises immunity levels makes exercise even more beneficial. When carefully planned, it can even prevent or reverse the need for some medications.

Daily stretching and low-impact aerobics plus two to three weekly sessions of strength training are recommended whether you have arthritis, hypertension, or osteoporosis along with your diabetes (get your doctor's approval). Depression best responds to group aerobics and weight workouts. Weight lifting, especially for women, seems to improve self-image as well as control depression.

Though walking is considered one of the best aerobic exercises, Dr. Joel Fuhrman contends that walking by itself is not sufficient exercise.* As a sole form of exercise, it can shift calcium and muscular development from the upper neck and spine to the legs and hips, leaving out the upper body, chest area (thoracic), and the cervical (neck) spine. He recommends including muscle-strengthening exercises along with walking.

Aerobics

Various sports may or may not be aerobic. Cross-country skiing is believed to be the exercise that is the most aerobic and helps balance and

---

*"Nutrition for Young and Old, Sick and Well" by A. Henderson-Boulter. Dr. Joel Fuhrman's approach to good health. In April 1998 issue of *Alternates and Complementary Therapies*, vol. 4, 2. Pages 122–127.

strengthen the body in more ways than any other type of exercise. Swimming comes in as a close second. (Note: overweight people should make sure that the pool water in which they are swimming is not cold. Apparently, swimming in cold water does not promote fat burning but promotes conservation of heat.) Volleyball, golf, tennis, and other stop/start sports are good for increasing activity levels but are not considered aerobic sports—unless you constantly keep moving in between swings.

Cross training is including two or more sports as part of an increased activity or exercise program. This type of training not only decreases boredom in doing the same thing day after day, but also involves various muscles, so that by the end of the week or month, most if not all the muscles are included. You need to pick and choose the exercise and activities best for you.

Swimming or water aerobics are particularly helpful for those who have difficulty walking or standing. Not only can breathing techniques be involved, but you can also improve muscle strength with the leg kicks and the arm movements. Move your head from side to side. Then move your head from front to back. Be sure to lift your arms high when reaching over for the next stroke versus using a bent-up elbow and arm. Keep your breathing even and deep, inhaling when your head is on its side and exhaling when it's below the surface of the water. For abdomen, buttock, chest, back, and shoulder strengthening, do the butterfly or free-style crawl. The breaststroke aids the chest and upper arms plus the thighs. The backstroke focuses on the thighs and upper arms.

For water aerobics, almost all of the stretches and bending movements may be carried out while standing in the water. The water supports the body so that gravity doesn't play as great a role in putting pressure on the feet and ankles as it would if you were standing and exercising on dry ground.

For starters, for the first five to ten minutes use easy strokes or, for water aerobics, move about in the water, gently moving your hands, arms, and legs. Work up to six laps or six cycles with each of the aforementioned strokes or water exercises. Change to rapid strokes in the pool or leg kicks while holding on to a kickboard or side of the pool. Cool down by doing exactly what you did in the warm-up.

Rope jumping is aerobic and has been developed as an art. Or join a health club and make new friends while toning and exercising at the same time. Or find your favorite trail to walk on. Determine your favorite exercise or sport. Or try something new.

Muscle Strengthening

For strengthening the muscles in various parts of your body, just "move" or exercise that part of the body. Some believe that if you exercise a certain body part, then you can reduce the fat of that body part. Not so. Fat, per se, is reduced throughout the whole body, but the muscles will be stronger in that part, resulting in more firmness in that area. For example, just standing up and sitting down without using your hands will increase the muscle fibers in your thighs.

If you desire upper body strength, use handheld weights to enhance these next exercises. Lying on your back, do a series of chest presses (bend the elbows and lower the weights to the shoulders and return). Or while still lying on your back move the weights from an outstretched, vertical position above your head to the floor on each side of your body. On standing, move the handheld weights from your sides in an arch up to the level of the shoulders, then move the weights, elbows bent, from the shoulder to the ceiling. Finally, hold the weights at your sides and bring them up to chest level, as if you were lifting a package. This is called the biceps curl.

While lying down, do abdominal crunches, remembering not only to do the ones where you lift the head off the floor but also raise the buttocks off the floor by tightening other muscles found in the abdomen. Then lie on your side, supported by the opposite hand placed on the floor, and move your outside leg forward, upward, and backward.

Firm up the lower body by doing squats, lunges, and steps. Squats may be done while resting the back against the wall or by just spreading the feet and bending the knees. Lunges are enhanced by holding weights in each hand (arms straight) and stepping forward with alternating right and left legs. A sturdy box or the first step on a stair can be used to alternately step up and down with each leg.

Use a chair to assist the hip for leg swings. It will help you balance as you stand on one or the other foot while you move your opposite leg backward, sideways, and forward. Swing your leg in each direction and to each side, ending up with full leg swings clockwise and counterclockwise.

Tension Relievers

For a short tension reliever and also to improve circulation to the extremities, including the head, try placing the palms of your hands on your eyes for a few minutes. Follow this by placing your hands on the back of your head and twisting your body right and left while still seated. While your hands are still placed on the back of your head, touch each elbow to the knee on the same side and then back into the resting position.

Now, place one hand up and over behind your head, touching your back, and place the other hand on the opposite elbow and stretch. Alternately, bend the knees to the chest, one at a time, while sitting on a chair. Next, stretch by placing your feet and hands as far back on each side of the chair as you are able. Complete this exercise with a moment of relaxation by again placing your palms on your eyes and breathing deeply.

There are a number of other body movements for tension relief that some consider exercises while others do not. These movements originated in other countries but are increasingly becoming popular in this country. Tai chi would be considered nonaerobic exercise by most, but in a sense, when the whole series of exercises are completed without stopping, it is as effective as low-impact aerobic might be.

Tai Chi

Tai chi is a sequence of martial art movements. It became a traditional Chinese exercise as a series of slow movements done in a continuous sequence. Tai chi has been documented to significantly lower the risk of dangerous falls among elderly men and women (*Journal of the American Geriatrics Society*). To flow through the movements takes concentration and produces a state of wakeful relaxation. It also helps with balance resulting in fewer falls and stronger bones.

Tai chi focuses on the inner life force known as *chi* (also spelled *qi*). The stance is balanced as you focus your weight through your lower back and down through your bent knees to the floor. A simple example of this is getting in a stance with feet placed out further than the shoulders, elbows bent, and feet parallel to each other. Gradually shift your weight to the right and then to the left, bending the knee a bit more when the weight is shifted to that side. You may learn Tai chi by reading books (most books have pictures or illustrations to show you what to do), viewing videotapes, or attending classes if available in your community. Or perhaps you would prefer Qigong—the exercise sequence developed for keeping the samurai healthy rather than preparing them for fighting (over two thousand years ago).

Qigong

Qigong is associated with energy balance. *Qi* (pronounced "chee") represents energy, which is found in heaven, on earth, and in every living thing (too much energy [positive] = too much yang; too little energy [negative] = too little yin). Gong stands for time and also for energy. Much of the practices were developed in India and then brought to China. Qigong meditations, carried on by those who taught these sequences, were used during the specified sequence of physical movements. There is a religious Qigong that kept the practices secret, and the non-religious Qigong which is used today. Its initial development was to improve the health of soldiers. It was also used in two martial styles; an external style and an internal style.

For help with balancing external energy (called Wai Dan), you concentrate your attention on your arms and legs. There are then many sets of practices that assist in this balancing process. Wai Dan Qigong builds up the energy in the arms and legs and then has energy flow to the organs. Wai Dan is mostly a physical process.

For internal exercise, Nei Dan must be learned from a master. Nei Dan involves energy that is built up in the body to then be spread out to the arms and the legs. To reach this higher level of processing, you must practice frequently—some say to the point of being a hermit. Nei Dan is mostly mental processing. If not done correctly, it can lead to mental problems such as depression, paranoia, etc. Wai Dan, however, is a safe practice.

As with any Tai chi or Qigong practice, no matter what type, you must remember the sequences of movements. This practice also involves relaxation; therefore, your way of breathing and state of calmness while you practice will lead to a relaxed body. The first level of relaxation that comes is postural. The second level is for the muscles and tendons. The third level is to reach the internal organs and bone marrow.

For these practices, you must be rooted or centered. Your body must be balanced. Breathing must be uniform and even. Deep breathing ability is a must. Regulating the mind requires thought stopping. Your mind is in the state of being separate from emotions.

It usually takes the most practice to reach this level where your state of being is separate from your emotions. When your mind is relaxed, the spirit is raised, the will is strengthened, and patience and endurance are increased.

Refer to the bibliography for information on Dr. Yang's book, *Eight Simple Qigong Exercises for Health,* and to obtain more details on the history and focus of health and description of these exercises.

Other Martial Arts

Try one of the other martial arts, recognizing that Tai chi was first established as such a practice. Kwando combines karate, kickboxing, and aerobics. Enter a dance class (that includes men, too) Movement and balance are part of each of these activities.

Many people are expressing an interest in Tae-Bo (www.taebo.com). It is popular because it combines the martial arts with low-impact aerobics. This total body workout was introduced by the former karate world champion Billy Blanks in the late 1980s. Participation in this activity can burn up to 700 calories an hour. It gives you an opportunity to work on coordination and balance, besides enhancing cardiovascular activity.

If balance alone is sought, try yoga.

YOGA

Like Tai chi, yoga works to unite mental, physical, and spiritual health. The exercises require controlled breathing and gentle stretching. You do not need to go along with its philosophy to participate in the activities involved. Yoga increases flexibility, strength, and stamina. It can assist in decreasing anxiety.

Classical yoga is divided into eight limbs, or paths, which include the ethical, the physical, the mental, the supramental, and god-consciousness. The first four limbs are centered on balancing the body and mind. The second four limbs focus on meditation.

Yoga means *union*. It is a Sanskrit word that has the same source as our word *yoke*. It represents an integration of the physical, mental, and spiritual energies for the enhancement of health.

Although first written down in the second century B.C., yoga has been practiced for over 6,000 years. Yoga calms and balances the body. Its advantage, in relation to outright exercise, is the attention to the endocrine and nervous systems by increasing circulation. For instance, the shoulder stand uses positive gravity to increase circulation in the thyroid gland, and improves the nervous system through correct breathing.

The more common yoga practices (*asanas*, which means *ease* in Sanskrit) are bhakti (for those seeking a pathway to God through love and devotion); hatha (the gentle yoga through the harmony of mind and body); jnana (the intellectually focused yoga using meditation and thought), karma (the yoga of service in action); kundalini (for awakening the primal forces through celibacy and turning one's sexual energy for the use of God); mantra (for affecting the body via the endocrine system through vibration energy with the use of sound); and raja (breathing for stilling the mind).

Hatha Yoga

Explore hatha yoga, as it is the most common form of yoga practiced. Hatha yoga has some major types or styles. These styles are Iyengar-style hatha yoga, which includes jumps and brisk movements; Integral yoga, which is a synthesis of traditional yogas using smooth, balanced movements; Vini yoga, with emphasis on breathing (*prana yama*); and Ashtanga yoga, also called Power yoga, which is for advanced students. The purpose is to detoxify the body through physical and psychological practices, which lead to alterations of your lifestyle and the elimination of waste products from the body. This includes practices that are meditative and therapeutic for the improvement of health and well-being while bringing the mind into a state of quiet energy flow. The Indian name for energy is *prana*. These activities are meant to aid in increasing *prana*.

Whatever breathing exercise is used, it must be sequentially flowing and regular. Regulated breathing goes along with meditation. The Mind-Body Institute at Harvard University documented how meditation practice can affect the breathing rate, the consumption of oxygen, the brain wave rhythms, and the flow of blood throughout the body.

Several other studies have demonstrated the effectiveness of yoga on pain alleviation, on intelligence and memory skills, on alleviating anxiety, on improving blood pressure and heart rate, and on enhanced metabolic and respiratory functions, to name a few.

OTHER CONSIDERATIONS

As noted earlier in this chapter, there are a variety of resources available through catalogs, health food stores, and department stores. When participating in an exercise program, remember that having diabetes is an opportunity, not an obstacle in starting a program. Learn to develop a safe and effective program in spite of having diabetes.

DIABETES MANAGEMENT

"Whenever any man [or woman] has done the best he
[or she] can, then that is all he [or she] can do."
—*Harry S Truman*

Insulin's role during exercise is to assist glucose transport and function in the working muscle. As a result, insulin inhibits the production of hepatic (liver) glucose, so the possibility of becoming hypoglycemic is greater during exercise.

In the nondiabetic, there is a decrease in the release of insulin during exercise. In someone who has Type 2 diabetes, it is possible to have an excess of insulin released. Be sure to monitor your blood sugar before and after exercising. If you exercise more than thirty to forty-five minutes, you may wish to take an extra snack.

Again, check your blood sugar before and after exercising. Standard reminders are, if the blood sugar is less than 60 mg/dL (3.3 mmol/L) then do not exercise. If the blood sugar is greater than 250 mg/dL (14 mmol/L), then check for ketones in the urine. A urine test with ketones indicates you should not exercise. If the urine does not have ketones, then proceed with your exercise plans. Do not exercise if the blood sugar is 300 + (16 mmol/L +).

Choose to exercise after a meal or snack. For high intensity exercise, snack every thirty to sixty minutes, usually using one to two points (75 to 140 calories) or fifteen to thirty grams of carbohydrate. Lower your previous dose of insulin if the exercise is to be prolonged and/or intensive, and don't inject into a muscle that will be purposely involved during an exercise or participatory sport.

Check with your diabetes health-care provider for specifics or refer to a number of resources such as a chart guide for adjusting insulin doses to duration and intensity of exercise (found in *Joslin's Diabetes Mellitus*). A reminder: these suggestions are only starting points. You need to adjust dosages to fit you and your particular exercise program.

Always keep glucose in some form and an extra snack with you when you're exercising, participating in a sport, or increasing your activity. An identification bracelet or necklace is also useful (identification in a purse or wallet might get lost). Having some money on hand would also be useful in case you need to call someone or to buy more food. (Note: 911 may be dialed toll-free.)

If you're serious about sports and exercise, join the International Diabetic Athletes Association (800-989-4322), or if sight is a problem, call (719-630-0422) for the United States Association for Blind Athletes.

Exercise might be considered a lost cause for some, but once you have started appropriately, it can give a lift to life and help balance the body. Even ten minutes a day has been found to be effective for weight control and is a good way to start.

Exercise is an especially preventive activity for children and adults. Overweight children are most likely to have—or in the future will have—Type 2 diabetes. Exercise is one of the best modalities to assist children not only to develop a balanced lifestyle, but also to increase the possibility of their being and staying healthy.

What is your decision? If you haven't made a decision to exercise, please take the time to do so. Decide (1) the frequency of exercise; (2) the pace—start out slow; (3) the time of day to exercise; and (4) the type of exercise. Warm up by stretches or slower activity. Keep pace with the type of sport or exercise or strengthening/toning activity. Cool down by doing stretches or a slower activity. You're on your way.

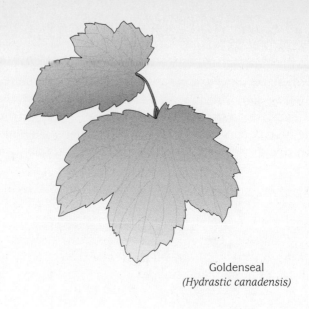

Goldenseal
(Hydrastic canadensis)

6

FOODS AND FOLLY

"If you eat junk food you'll feel junky." —*Guthrie and Guthrie*

Delores had been sick with a cough, sore throat, sneezing, and nasal discharge since the month of January. Now it was May. Her blood sugars had been elevated, but were only semicontrolled. She would have only a day or two of rest and then come down with another of the above symptoms.

She went to her traditional physician and was told she was just under a lot of stress and to take it easy. She decided to go to an alternative therapist and found that she had elevated vitamin B_3, (which is more typical in Type 2 diabetes, a finding reported by a Banting award winner—the highest award given in the field of diabetes research), but very low B_1, B_6, and vitamin C levels. She was to receive intravenous mega-doses of vitamin C (15 gms) with magnesium once a week for five weeks along with replacement therapy of the vitamins B_1 and B_6. Each week, the symptoms took a few days longer to return.

Placebo effect or not, after the fifth treatment she was symptom free. Daily timed release of 500 mg of vitamin C (or by food) with magnesium (less chance of a kidney stone problem) have kept her in a state where she has not had symptoms or been ill for three years. Along with normalized B_1 and B_6 levels, she was able to maintain her glucose levels with appropriate food choices.

GENERAL NUTRITION

That old saying "You are what you eat" is becoming more true each day. As more information is available, some of which contradicts other information, people who attempt to eat healthful foods are bombarded by the idea of "living to eat" rather than "eating to live." In spite of controversy and conflicting information, your goals should be to aim for the big picture, which is the attainment and maintenance of a healthy weight. A healthy weight and as active a lifestyle as possible promote better blood glucose control. The better the blood sugars are controlled, the less the risk of developing complications too often associated with diabetes (such as eye disease, kidney disease, nerve disease, and heart disease).

Many studies have now concluded that all people do not fit into the mold of having a "normal" weight for their height. Genetic structure and social expectations have won out. It is more difficult for some to lose weight than for others. In some cultures, mild to moderate obesity is considered a sign of beauty, wealth, or even health, and the desire to lose weight isn't there.

Weighing this against what the media say you can or should eat is often confusing. The vitamins and minerals stated to promote good health (the Recommended Dietary Allowance's [RDA's] guidelines for healthy food intake) are obtained if various foods are eaten on a daily or weekly basis. More and more advertisements entice you to take this vitamin, that mineral, or this great herb. To lessen this confusion, this chapter shall provide the normal nutritional guidelines to attain weight loss and keep it off, as well as information and principles in choosing the use of specific vitamins and minerals. In chapter 7, information and principles will be given on the use of herbal-based products.

Normal Nutrition

What is normal "nutrition"? What might be normal for you might not be normal for me. As a whole, the RDA presents the findings of current research. It does not address individual needs. The RDA's 1990s recommendations indicate a lesser need for the use of supplemental vitamins and minerals. The pharmaceutical industries that promote such products disputed these findings, as it meant that fewer people would buy their products. They fought the report of these new findings.

Research also revealed that what the body doesn't use, it releases from the body in its waste products. This is especially true of water-soluble products. This information was given to protect the consumer from ingesting unnecessary pills, with the message that all the excess, unneeded vitamins and minerals were doing was "feeding the fish." There was a push, and still is to some extent, to have the Food and Drug Administration (FDA) regulate the use of vitamins and minerals and herbs by requiring a prescription from a health professional in order to buy them. But the public didn't want to have the FDA or any other organization dictate what it could or could not choose. The first bill introduced into Congress had problems. Others are being written.

Some people process vitamins faster than others. An example is the use of vitamin C in the body. When people are highly stressed, it appears that vitamin C is more rapidly excreted from the body. Rates of speed and/or absorption factors influence the effectiveness of other vitamins and minerals while each vitamin and mineral has a specific purpose or purposes in the body. (See appendix B for a listing of vitamins and minerals.)

It would be helpful if it were possible to have an inexpensive way of analyzing the blood for the presence of these sources of assistance, but it would leave out of the loop the presence or lack of vitamins and minerals found in the cells. Until there is a method of letting you know what your body needs presently and what you lack in the way of vitamins and minerals, nutrition will not be an exact science.

General recommendations for eating guidelines are now presented to the public through the use of the Food Guide Pyramid. Controversy even exists as to what should be placed where on this diagram.

There is little debate about placing fats and sugars at the top of the pyramid. Even people of differing viewpoints agree that small quantities of these foods are recommended.

Underlying the top of the pyramid section is the directive to eat meat and dairy products in certain amounts (please refer to the diagram below). Fruits and vegetables follow on the third level, and breads and grains are found at the bottom level of the pyramid.

The biggest controversy concerns these last two levels. A group states that fruits and vegetables need to be eaten in greater quantities than breads and grains and, therefore, should form the foundation for this pyramid. The pyramid for the elderly has as its base eight glasses of water per day.

If you are a vegetarian you could be of the type who omits just animal meats or who believes that all products from animals should be eliminated from the diet. Protein may be obtained through eating certain vegetables and by eating nuts. A complete protein from vegetable sources requires two to three specific vegetables (such as corn and beans and/or brown rice) to be eaten at the same meal or within a short period of time.

Breads, grains, and pastas form a group of foods that obese individuals are often told to omit in their meal plan. Whatever the omission, if a vitamin or mineral is not obtained by eating certain foods, then there is a need for a synthetic replacement.

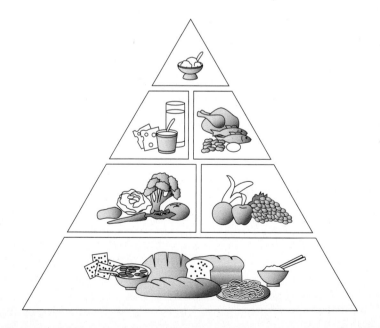

Diet Types Overview

Types of diets other than the USRDA focus on balancing the types of foods available according to either religious beliefs, ethical considerations, supplementary needs, and desire for weight reduction. Jewish dietary laws, especially Orthodox, are the basis for extremely rigorous guidelines, such as the nonuse of pork and the noncombination of meat with dairy products.

Christian groups vary. Some omit tea, coffee, and alcohol or any other stimulants, like the Mormons and Seventh Day Adventists. Many Catholics still eat fish on Friday, even though this restriction was lifted by Pope John XXIII. And many Christian groups restrict eating meat during Lent.

The Koran prohibits the use of alcoholic drinks and the eating of pork.

Macrobiotic diets are a system based on yin- and yang-type foods that are mostly cooked. This type of diet was originally found in Asian homes. Yin foods tend to be hot foods, more frequently grown in hot climates. Yang foods are sour and salty, being grown in cold, usually wet, areas. It is believed that when the intake of yin and yang foods are not in balance, the person becomes ill. Five percent or less of this diet includes fruits. Dairy and egg-based foods are avoided. Baked goods and pastas are avoided. Any foods related to the nightshade plant (such as potatoes, tomatoes, and yams) are avoided. Spices are considered too stimulating.

Today, people following a macrobiotic diet often combine it with fasting, meditation, and prayer. The American Medical Association objected to the macrobiotic analysis of foods and the lack of inclusion of some foods, especially protein foods, and considered the purist form as actually dangerous. Vitamins and minerals are found to be the least available, protein next, followed by fats and the major composition of the diet, complex carbohydrates. Along with protein deficiency, there may be the added problem of high salt and overacidity.

Vegetarianism goes back as far as the Greeks in the sixth century B.C. The most famous vegetarians were Plato and Pythagoras. It was further developed around the middle of the 1800s. Not eating meat was based on the ethical principles of not eating anything considered flesh, but it allows milk, milk products, and eggs (ovo-lacto vegetarianism). Lacto-vegetarians permit milk and milk products but not eggs. Veganism avoids all flesh or flesh-associated (e.g., egg) products, even honey (for some). They may even go as far as the nonuse of anything made with products from animals.

Vitamin B_{12} deficiency is a potential problem when following this program. Then there are the go-betweens, such as those who don't eat meat but do eat fish. Various groups choose to be vegetarians, such as the Hindus, for religious purposes or the natives who live in the Andes, who basically have only corn and beans plus a very high-yield wheat protein to eat.

For a complete protein, the vegetarian must combine a variety of vegetables, grains and legumes, or nuts and legumes, or vegetables and milk, or eggs. When vegetarians chose foods wisely, it is has been found that they can obtain the essential nutrients the body needs.

Food combining is something promoted by naturopaths and some homeopaths. The theory is to eat certain foods and combine or not combine them with certain other foods for the best digestion. Fruits are eaten alone. A sweet fruit is not eaten with an acid fruit. Melon fruits are eaten alone. Protein foods (requiring an acid medium for digestion) are not eaten with starches, such as breads that need an alkaline digestive medium. Protein foods could be eaten with green vegetables, or green vegetables could be combined with starches. Milk is only used in foods and not as a drink.

Food rotation has each food in the diet eaten only in one day out of four to minimize the allergic "stimulus" of each food.

An acid-alkaline-balanced diet is one in which the foods eaten are more alkaline (some fruits and all vegetables) to pair with the more alkaline elements of the body (that is, 70 percent of foods eaten are alkaline in nature).

Various Diet Programs

It seems that a new approach to eating is reported nearly every day. The following programs only represent some of what is available. The length of the presentation of a specific approach does not indicate approval, but each topic is discussed in such a way to help you decide which program is most beneficial for you. The following programs are placed in no particular sequence.

The Pritikin Diet

Nathan Pritikin, the founder of the center that bears his name, cured his own heart and blood vessel disease through diet. Basically, he cut down on fats, salt, animal protein, and sugar and increased his intake of complex carbohydrates such as beans, grains, and corn, and the use of fresh fruits.

The Pritikin diet includes 10 percent of total calories from fat and 15 percent from protein with 75 percent to 80 percent carbohydrate. This diet has been found useful for a variety of people. Cholesterol is restricted to less than 100 mgs after the participant is on the "regression" diet of eight low-calorie meals a day (1,000 calories for women, 1,200 calories for men). It is expected that a person participating in this program will produce a lot of intestinal gas (a result of the greater than 35 grams/day of fiber), but be healthier. Alcohol is excluded. Protein content is somewhat low. The Pritikin Center in California includes classes on nutrition and lifestyle changes. Food preparation is also a part of the course as are exercise, calming activities, and quiet time.

The meat allowed must be lean (only 4 ounces per day allowed), or skinless if chicken, or fish. Only the whites of eggs are included. Since this is an extremely low-fat diet, problems with deficiencies in vitamins A, D, E, and K plus some essential fatty acids are of concern, especially if this diet is used over a prolonged period of time. A number of programs knowledgeable about these factors will use the diet to treat the illness and then follow with a mainstream type of diet.

The Ornish Diet

The Ornish diet has been described by some as being similar to the Pritikin Diet (that is, 10 percent fat, 10 percent low protein, 75 percent to 80 percent carbohydrate). Seeds and nuts are excluded. No meat, poultry, egg yolks, and alcohol are allowed, and they are replaced by fiber and complex carbohydrates. Both meal plans have shown good results when it comes to controlling and reversing heart disease. You may also participate in this program on-site and learn more of the details about cooking, eating, and changing your lifestyle. Whole foods are encouraged. As in the Pritikin program, amounts of complex carbohydrates are not restricted, which leads to better compliance.

Dr. Dean Ornish, director of the Life Choice Program (in Sausalito, California) and others from the University of California, studied how less than 10 percent fat intake along with stress management, exercise, and smoking cessation affected the blood vessels in the body, especially those already damaged by poor eating and living habits. In one year, they were able to show that 91 percent of their population had less frequent chest pain along with a reduction of cholesterol levels. Others have been able to duplicate their findings.

Others, such as Dr. Meyer Friedman and his coworkers, found that over a five-year period, people following the Ornish dietary program had only half the number of heart attacks as compared to those who followed their usual dietary intake, smoked, and didn't exercise.

Both the Ornish and Pritikin diets are safe so long as there is 10 percent or more complete protein available to the consumer on a daily basis.

The Atkins Diet

Dr. Atkins's *New Diet Revolution,* written by a physician whose first book about low-carbohydrate dieting was a multimillion-dollar best-seller in 1972, continues to treat his patients today with a low-carbohydrate diet. The Atkins diet really consists of four phases or four diet plans along with comprehensive vitamin and nutrient supplementation. Phase one is the induction diet; phase two—ongoing weight loss; phase three—premaintenance; and phase four—maintenance diet.

Dr. Atkins calls the first phase of his diet program the induction diet. It is a corrective diet whose primary purpose is to correct, as expeditiously as possible, an unbalanced metabolism. It is designed to create ketosis/lipolysis to cause weight loss. Ketosis means that you are burning your fat stores for energy. This phase lasts fourteen days. The induction diet "rules" consist of 20 grams or less of carbohydrate intake per day. He encourages the use of a carbohydrate gram counter to know how to calculate and stay within the 20 gram carbohydrate limit.

Dietary supplements are a very important part of the Atkins diet. Dr. Atkins reported that the small amount of vegetables in the induction phase of his diet will not provide enough nutrients and that most people's vitamin and mineral reserves are depleted before the diet. He recommends supplements for everyone. As for the induction phase, Dr. Atkins cautions that if you have a serious disease, this should only be done under the supervision of a physician, and that this diet is not appropriate for people with severe kidney disease or for pregnant women.

The ongoing weight loss diet incorporates the "Critical Carbohydrate Level for Losing." He advises doing this with caution, eating low-carbohydrate vegetables, nuts, and other foods to enhance your diet but still remain in the ketosis/lipolysis mode. This phase of the diet usually consists of 15 to 60 grams of carbohydrate a day, depending on your metabolism, and can take a few weeks to a few months.

The premaintenance phase is next, when you have only a few more pounds to lose. It is a way to gradually move toward the maintenance diet. Dr. Atkins sees this as one phase that prepares you for your lifetime dietary habit.

The maintenance diet is very individualized regarding carbohydrate intake. The guiding question at this stage is "what level of carbohydrate consumption do I feel best on?" This will vary from person to person, from about 25 to 90 grams a day. Dr. Atkins found that your best carbohydrate level is the one you can be happiest on without weight regain. A recent research project done at the Atkins Center shows results suggesting that a high-protein low-carbohydrate diet with nutritional supplementation can be useful to reduce several cardiovascular risk factors including weight, blood sugar, and lipid parameters in obese patients with Type 2 diabetes.

The Bernstein Approach

Another program was developed by Dr. Richard Bernstein, the author of *The Laws of Small Numbers*. He is a physician who has had Type 1 diabetes since age twelve. His health continued to fail despite following the recommended diabetes protocol for over twenty years. In 1969 he developed a method of normalizing his blood sugars, which allowed him to reverse some of the complications he had developed. He entered medical school at age forty-five so he could publish his work and help other people with diabetes. Like Dr. Atkins, he also recommends a low-carbohydrate diet. Unlike Dr. Atkins, he recommends controlled fat intake.

Bernstein presents a very important concept in his diabetes treatment. Big intakes make big mistakes; small intakes make small mistakes. For someone with diabetes, the name of the game in achieving blood sugar normalization is predictability. It's difficult to use medications safely unless you can predict their effect. The same with food; you can't normalize blood sugar unless you can predict the effects of what you are eating. *If you can't predict your blood sugar level, you can't predict your insulin needs.* If the kinds of foods you're eating give you unpredictable blood sugar levels, then it is impossible to normalize blood sugars.

His book provides what needs to be learned to be able to predict blood sugar levels accurately. Here is where "the law of small numbers" is important. As for diet, he says carbohydrates affect blood sugar the most, so he recommends a low-carbohydrate diet. He states that the problem with the American Diabetes Association (ADA) diet is the big inputs of food (carbohydrates) that raise blood sugar the most. Dr. Bernstein's diet plan of low carbohydrates aims at keeping the blood sugar rise at about one-tenth of the ADA diet, 10 to 20mg/dL. The key is to eat foods that will affect your blood sugar in a very small way. Stay with low levels of carbohydrates. In addition, stick with foods that will make you feel satisfied without causing huge swings in blood sugar. Essential to "obeying" the laws of small numbers is to eat only a small amount of slow-acting carbohydrates when you eat carbohydrates, and to eat no fast-acting carbohydrates. Even the slowest-acting carbohydrates can outpace injected insulin or one's own insulin release if consumed in greater amounts than recommended.

Dr. Bernstein's basic approach in negotiating a meal plan is to first set the carbohydrate limits for each meal. Then he asks his patient to tell him how many ounces of protein it will take to make him/her satisfied. He usually advises his patients to restrict their carbohydrate intake at breakfast to about 6 grams of slow-acting carbohydrates, 12 grams for lunch, and 12 grams for supper. Ideally, your blood sugar should be the same after eating as it was before. If your blood sugar increases by more that 20 mg/dL after a meal, even if it eventually drops to your target value, either the meal content should be changed or blood sugar lowering medications should be used before eating.

He has demonstrated in his clinic that this approach can work if you are or are not on insulin or other medications. Dr. Bernstein feels this is an effective way of maintaining a more constant blood sugar.

The Eades Approach

Dr. Michael R. Eades and Dr. Mary Dan Eades are the two physicians (specializing in weight loss) who wrote *Protein Power*. The authors have unique medical interests: Michael, paleopathology and biochemistry; his wife, Mary Dan, anthropology and has published a book on eating disorders. They worked for years with patients who had illnesses related to disordered insulin metabolism. With further studies, they came to the conclusion that excess carbohydrate consumption isn't good. But they did not know why. They were physicians, so they understood that the immediate effect of carbohydrate consumption was an elevated blood glucose, then an elevated insulin level. At about the same time, other researchers were finding a relation between elevated insulin levels and heart disease, high blood pressure, and diabetes, the common diseases of modern man. They concluded that by decreasing carbohydrate intake rather than increasing it, their patients would be better off. They then looked at this theory from a biochemical perspective and found that it worked. They do advise medical supervision if a person is over 20 percent overweight, or has a serious health problem like diabetes.

The Protein Power Program can be summarized as follows. First, determine protein needs (a tool is provided to calculate these needs).

Choose fish, poultry, meat, low-fat cheese, eggs, and tofu for protein needs. Add 30 grams or less of carbohydrate, divided throughout the day, for Phase I intervention (if needing to lose a lot of fat/or correct a health problem) or 55 grams or less for Phase II (if wanting to lose a little fat, recompose the body's lean-to-fat ratio, or improve general health).

Fiber can be subtracted from the carbohydrate to find the effective carbohydrate count. They say to try to get 25 grams of fiber per day by choosing from leafy green vegetables, tomatoes, peppers, avocados, broccoli, cucumber, mushrooms, and salads. Sugar, starches, and starchy vegetables such as potatoes, corn, and beans (except green beans) will be temporarily eliminated. They do recommend healthful fats, nut oils, avocado, and butter because the body will use the fat for "fuel." If a dessert is desired, a low-carbohydrate fruit or sugar-free Jell-O are good choices.

A minimum of eight glasses of water a day is encouraged. Other fluid intake may include a glass of wine, lite beer, or diet sodas. Artificial sweeteners are okay, but in moderation. Some added tips mentioned were to eat three meals a day and have snacks available to prevent hunger. If snacks are eaten, these carbohydrates should be included in the daily carbohydrate count. They recommend a good quality multi-vitamin supplement along with at least 90 mg of potassium. This diet is aimed at correcting the underlying insulin resistance by lowering the abnormally elevated blood sugar levels. They state that even those with Type 1 diabetes can markedly lower their insulin doses and attain much better control over their blood sugars with this plan, but *only under the supervision of a physician.*

The Schwarzbein Diet

Dr. Diana Schwarzbein, a physician specializing in endocrinology and metabolism, wrote *The Schwarzbein Principle* and speaks about her earlier frustration with the high-carbohydrate, low-fat diet, and the current "standard of care." Her patients didn't do well, gained weight, had difficulty regulating blood sugars, blood pressure, and had the complications of diabetes. Before incorporating the low-carbohydrate diet, she too was taught that the link between elevated insulin levels, diabetes, obesity, and heart disease was genetic. Wanting to help her patients, she realized that the carbohydrates were raising their blood sugars, which in turn increased insulin levels, so she started to try a low-carbohydrate diet but still using low fat. Many of her patients started eating higher fat foods, like red meats, cheeses, eggs, and these patients did very well. It seemed that the patients that "cheated the most, did the best." With further study she learned that insulin resistance is related to the aging process, and degenerative diseases.

Dr. Schwarzbein describes Type 2 diabetes as a metabolic continuum involving both insulin and blood sugar levels. Since her main goal is to decrease insulin levels, Dr. Schwarzbein does not advocate oral hypoglycemic agents that stimulate the release of insulin. She prescribes a treatment program combining regular exercise, a cutback in stimulants and other drugs, and a diet consisting of lower carbohydrates. She asks that blood sugars be checked before and one hour after meals to evaluate the numbers and adjust carbohydrates accordingly.

Dr. Schwarzbein prescribes two different nutritional programs. One is for healing, the other for maintenance. The nutritional healing program eliminates all sugars, chemicals, and drugs. Also, it reduces carbohydrate consumption while including needed proteins and fats. She observes that if this approach is used, then insulin resistance is reversed. She concluded that by decreasing carbohydrates you can begin to reverse insulin resistance, and you are then on your way to reversing accelerated metabolic aging.

The basic guidelines for this healing program include: eating all the good fats and proteins your body needs, eating a variety of nonstarchy vegetables, eating carbohydrates according to your current metabolism and activity level, avoiding manmade carbohydrates, caffeine, artificial sweeteners, processed packaged foods, stimulants, and over-the-counter medication. She wants each person to ask his/her physician if he/she can stop any prescription medications. (She notes that any drug has the potential to have an adverse effect at the cellular level.)

The Schwarzbein Nutritional Maintenance Program follows the healing program and is for people who are already healthy and want to stay that way. The maintenance program is the same as the healing program except you do not decrease your carbohydrates below your metabolic needs. Dr. Schwarzbein's diet is a balanced diet of protein and fats, with carbohydrate consumption appropriate to each person's metabolic and activity level.

The Steward Approach

Dr. Steward, a scientist, and three physicians, one of whom is an endocrinologist, developed this approach for meal planning. The main gist of their book, entitled *Sugar Busters,* is to avoid refined foods, such as cake and pie, most specifically to avoid foods with a high glycemic potential or index. In understanding how the metabolism of carbohydrates relates to the recommendations for good nutrition and weight loss, it is very important to think of carbohydrates in terms of how much of a peak or rise of glucose they can cause in the body when eaten. This can more simply be called the glycemic potential, which varies for different types of carbohydrates, and in more scientific terms can be called the glycemic index. The higher the rise, the higher the glycemic potential or index.

The authors do not really consider this diet to be low carbohydrate, but rather lower than the ADA recommends. *Sugar Busters* recommends 40 percent carbohydrates (with a low glycemic index), 30 percent fat (less than 10 percent saturated fat, 20+ percent polyunsaturated/monounsaturated fat), and 30 percent protein. The authors say this diet works because in the diabetes state, the pancreas does not make enough insulin or the body cannot respond to the insulin that is made efficiently (insulin resistance). Most often the problem is insulin resistance, and in this case the body needs more insulin than someone who does not have diabetes to keep blood sugar in a normal range. Following the *Sugar Busters* diet should cause a lower rise in blood glucose, therefore less insulin needs.

In summary, they say their concept is based on using good nutrition to effect a positive influence on insulin and glucagon secretion. This is achieved by eating food combinations that are properly composed of natural unrefined sugars, whole, unprocessed vegetables and fruits, lean meats, fiber, and if used, alcohol (in moderation).

The authors also recommend professional advice before changing to their diet because following the *Sugar Busters* diet has decreased the need for medication, be it pills or insulin.

The Method of Dr. Sears

Dr. Barry Sears, Ph.D. and Nobel Prize–winning researcher, wrote *The Zone* and (the more easily readable) *Mastering the Zone* in hopes of helping people understand and achieve a way for permanent weight loss while reaching peak mental and physical performance. What is the Zone? Expressed simply, it's the metabolic state in which the body works at peak efficiency.

Dr. Sears talks about insulin and glucagon, but also about other not-so-familiar hormones. These hormones are called eicosanoids. If hormones such as insulin and glucagon control blood sugar, what controls the hormones? The answer is eicosanoids. These are the body's super-hormones. Mysterious and fleeting but all-powerful, eicosanoids are made by every living cell in the human body. They're the molecular glue that holds the human body together. Eicosanoids are the most powerful biological agents known to man. If you can control eicosanoids, you'll open the door to the Zone.

Dr. Sears does not consider the Zone diet to be a low-carbohydrate diet but rather a protein-adequate, low-fat, moderate-carbohydrate program. If we want to reap the benefits from "living in the Zone" we will need to think of eating as something as powerful as taking medicine. When food is broken down into its basic components (glucose, amino acids, and fatty acids) and assimilated, it has a more powerful impact on your body—and your health—than any drug your doctor could ever prescribe.

The Zone diet is not a calorie counting diet. It is based on a ratio of protein to carbohydrate as close to 0.75 as possible each time you eat. The rules to meet this ratio are as follows. The first step is to calculate your own unique protein requirement. In his book he provides a tool to do so. Once you know your protein requirement, you build on this. First of all, spread the amount throughout the day, over three meals and two snacks. He tries to make this calculation easier by using what he calls a macro nutrient block method. A protein block consists of 7 grams of protein. For example, if your total protein requirement for the day is 75 grams, you would require 11 protein blocks per day (rounding the number off to the nearest whole number). To spread this throughout the day you would eat three protein blocks at each meal and one at each of the two snacks. To stay in the Zone, Dr. Sears recommends that you go no longer than five hours without a meal or snack.

The next part of calculating the Zone diet is to add carbohydrates. For every protein block you eat, you should eat one carbohydrate block. A carbohydrate block consists of 9 grams of "favorable" carbohydrate. This will maintain the protein-to-carbohydrate ratio of 0.75. Favorable carbohydrates usually have a low glycemic index—they enter the bloodstream slowly, raise blood sugar levels slowly, and produce a moderate insulin response. This means they maintain a favorable balance of eicosanoids that keeps you in the Zone.

As for saturated fat, he also recommends keeping these to a minimum, but for a different reason. He says these raise insulin levels. The "good" fats he recommends are monounsaturated fats, which are found in olive oil, canola oil, olives, macadamia nuts, and avocados.

The conclusion from the results of a recent clinical trial showed that a protein-adequate, carbohydrate-moderate, low-fat, calorie-restricted diet can be integrated readily into the lifestyle of patients with Type 2 diabetes. Dr. Sears has found this integration of eating according to his program to provide highly significant clinical improvement within six weeks, such as a 23 percent decrease in insulin levels, a hemoglobin A_{1c} decrease to 7 percent, a 14 percent decrease in triglycerides, and a 26 percent decrease in the ratio of triglycerides to high density lipoprotein.

CONCLUDING THOUGHTS ON PROGRAMS

In conclusion, the authors of these books have some common points. Compared with the dietary recommendation of the American Diabetes Association's low-fat, low-protein, high-carbohydrate diet, these programs present a diet lower in carbohydrates and higher in protein as a valid approach to the prevention of Type 2 diabetes and treatment of Types 1 and 2 diabetes.

If you are interested in following one of these programs, there is one other major consideration besides coordinating this change with your health professional. Be sure the functioning of your liver and kidneys are adequate. Liver and kidney disease could bring about problems that challenge the body's mechanisms to handle waste products when faced with high-protein loads.

A high fluid intake is recommended with any high-protein meal plan. A condition called azotemia, or protein the blood can be an outcome. Close physician supervision is a must. Again, the principles should be:

1. Use moderation in all things.
2. Listen to your body.
3. Ask questions.
4. Be aware of the effect of the meal program on any diabetes complication and vice versa.

OBESITY

"The (person) who removes a mountain begins by carrying
away small stones." —*Chinese proverb*

Obesity is defined as having a body mass index (BMI) above 30. Your BMI is calculated by dividing your weight in pounds by your height in inches squared, and that number is multiplied by 705. Consider a BMI of under 20 as underweight; 20 to 26 as healthy weight; 27 to 30 as overweight, 31 to 39 as very overweight or obese; and above 40 as extremely overweight or extremely obese. The disease risk is higher if the BMI is 35 to 40 or more.

One more method is to multiply your weight by 703 and your height in inches by itself. Then divide the weight result by the height result for the BMI.

Another system is measuring your waist at the narrowest point and dividing this number by the measurement of your hips at the widest point. For women, the number of concern is greater than 0.80 or for men, if this number is greater than 1.0. The health risk is higher if the number is 1.0 or higher.

Another way to define obesity is if you have a percentage of body fat above the acceptable level, which should range from 18 to 23 percent in men and 25 to 30 percent in women. Men are able to lose weight faster than women as they burn 10 to 20 percent more calories than women do in the resting state. Percent body fat is more of a predictor of problems than just being overweight (i.e., muscle mass weighs more than fat mass; weight that is 10 percent above the upper limit of normal indicates being overweight; 20 percent above indicates obesity). Those 30 to 40 billion fat cells can be filled to the point where not only the waist size increases, but the interior organs are also crowded. Yes, fat cells are present not only under the skin's surface but also internally, especially in the peritoneal (inside your abdomen) area.

Obesity primarily occurs when more is eaten than is expended as energy or released from the body as a waste product. (Though genetics may or may not lead to obesity, it can make you more susceptible to weight gain.) If you have Type 2 diabetes, especially when you are producing excess insulin, you seem to just look at food and gain weight. If you have Type 1 or Type 2 diabetes mellitus and have normalized your blood glucose levels, the ease with which you can gain weight is remarkable. Many people forget that the major use of insulin is to assist in storing food. This is called the feast or famine principle. This relates back to "caveman" days. When you feasted, your body stored the excess calories as fat. You used these excess fat calories during the times when food was not readily available (fasting state).

Obesity as an Addictive Disease

Obesity is considered an addictive disease by some. Overeaters Anonymous recognizes that when food is eaten for the wrong reason and in increasing amounts, its use parallels the same pattern as the person addicted to drugs and alcohol. Bariatrists, or physicians who specialize in the field of obesity, recognize obesity as a disease. Diseases require treatment. Medications have been and are being developed to treat obesity, and like hypertension, the bariatrists feel they need to be taken for a lifetime.

People with Type 2 diabetes often produce excess insulin. Having excess insulin makes you feel hungry. The major treatment for hunger is to eat. We now know that if you have the genetics to be overweight, even starting as a child, you may also have the genetics for Type 2 diabetes.

As noted before, the major purpose of insulin is a storage hormone. The more you eat and the less active you become, the more weight you gain. If you have become metabolically conservative (eating as little as 500 to 900 calories a day) without an increase in activity, even eating slightly more food means more pounds gained.

Barbara Harris's work on primates and obesity demonstrates this very clearly. Her research included various types of diets. One group of animals was left to eat as much of this "diet" as desired. The other group was given only a controlled amount of food each day as dictated by that particular diet plan. You can guess which group of animals gained weight.

Whatever Dr. Harris tried—varying diet plans or diet programs—the same result occurred. When activity level of the animals remained the same, the more they ate, even of nourishing foods, the more weight was gained.

This does not support the quick fix that most diet plans promote. It does make it plain and simple: if you eat more and don't burn the calories off by activity or exercise, you gain weight.

Losing Weight

> "It's kind of fun to do the impossible." —*Walt Disney*

Just start in a positive vein by working on shrinking your stomach. Removing a few teaspoons to tablespoons of each serving should help accomplish this.

Activity and exercise play a large part in this picture. For example, one slice of cheese pizza, which is equal to about 153 calories, takes about seventeen minutes of cycling to burn off. If you are sedentary (watching TV all the time), then there is more of a chance that the unused calories will be deposited in the fat cells. And alternately, if you diet to the extent that your body becomes metabolically conservative (thinking the body is fasting) and then you eat a calculated number of calories for your height and weight, you will find yourself gaining weight. This weight gain often occurs with eating fewer calories than actually indicated for height and weight.

The three considerations for loss of weight control are: (1) one and a half slices of bread per day (or the equivalent, for example, one and a half cups of mashed potatoes) intake over what you need will result in a pound of weight gained in one month; (2) exceeding 30 calories per pound (range 25 to 40 calories per pound) when prepubescent (before the start of the development of adult physical characteristics) versus 30 calories per kilogram (range 20 to 35 per kilogram) when postpubescent (once hair growth, breast, and genital growth have been completed), and (3) if more calories are taken in than energy expended, weight gain will occur. (2.2 pounds = 1 kilogram.)

The first indicates that it doesn't take much food volume to lead to weight gain if the activity level does not match the increased food intake. The second wisely demonstrates that the person who has developed adult characteristics needs less total food caloric intake; in fact, about half as much food is needed. And, the third is the vicious cycle where the more you eat, and the less active you are, or if you are less active but are still eating the same amount, weight gain is still the outcome.

To stop this cycle, the opposite must be achieved. Just restricting food intake is not enough. Increased activity or exercise daily or every other day is a must. What you choose to do for activity and exercise is up to you, and can be as varied as you would like it to be (as described in chapter 5). Getting a program that is coordinated with your ability and expectations is the major problem. People wish to lose weight "yesterday!"

If you wish to lose weight, you must eat less but include an adequate amount of food for repair of tissues and for energy for daily tasks. Accompanying this food intake must be a level of energy expenditure that not only assists in developing cardiovascular health, but also aids in muscle stretching and toning. Any diet will work if these two principles are carried out: (1) eating the amount of food needed (or slightly less) for energy and daily needs, and (2) keeping or increasing the activity or exercise level.

Starting such a program is a major problem. But doing it with outside support has been shown to be very effective, e.g., Weight Watchers, Overeaters Anonymous, Jenny Craig Program, or just the next-door neighbor. Maintaining a program for two years or longer is a must.

A visit with a dietitian is most useful. She or he will help to design a food intake program that is specific for your needs and your height versus your weight. This professional can also give you guidance on your activity program, or you could go to the expense of hiring a personal weight trainer or working with an exercise specialist. Diabetes educators may be of assistance in this preplanning process.

You need to determine what you are eating now and find the caloric level that would give you slow weight loss (one half to one pound per week for women and one to two pounds a week for men). This should be accompanied by a gradual increase in activity or exercise.

Blood glucose measurements will provide the information needed to change diabetes medication when such a need arises. For instance, with weight loss, people with Type 2 diabetes would need less medication, especially if the food intake is decreased, the activity level is increased, or both, and the blood glucose levels at the start of the program have been normal most of the time.

Weight loss centers may be useful, but they can cost from a one-time fee for membership per year (plus cost for products and manuals or other reading material) up to $4,000 for a program one week or longer at a health center. Many programs have specific days or weeks for people with diabetes. Other programs focus on general nutrition and health education. Generally, the programs meet the needs of a person with Type 2 diabetes, but someone with Type 1 diabetes could also benefit, especially if the program is coordinated with the person's diabetes specialist.

Whatever the program, focus on eating whole foods (such as fresh fruits and vegetables rather than canned) that contain more complex nutrients (for example, an orange provides vitamin C, carotene, calcium, and simple sugars).

The Hardest Part

Keeping up this regimen of diet and exercise is the hardest part. Any excuse can become a means to interrupt the program, and the body has a mean streak. It has a tendency, in one to two years, if the program is interrupted, of returning the person to the same weight with usually a few pounds added to boot. The behavioral change needed for attaining and maintaining any such program is really not considered successful unless two or more years have been reached where weight gain has not been the outcome.

Keeping your emotions on an even keel assists you in maintaining this weight loss. As was true during the weight loss period, so it is true once you have achieved the desired weight loss. Sadness or anger are key emotions that lead most people to indulge in "self-pity parties."

You need to preplan what you are going to do if you see yourself relapsing, such as getting back into the "old" way of eating or acting.

Check in on Merlene and Dave Miller's book, *Reversing the Weight Gain Spiral*. Merlene Miller also is an author on other relapse prevention books as well as a book about addictions, *Learning to Live Again*. These books and others will help you to find more ways to take out your anger or depression rather than on the misuse of food. Preplanning is one of the most useful tools.

Weight Loss Drugs

> "Our greatest glory is not in never failing, but in rising
> up every time we fail." —*Ralph Waldo Emerson*

Weight loss drugs should be avoided and only used if absolutely needed. Behavioral change is the "least toxic" (no side effect such as high blood pressure) way to proceed. But if you have tried everything, new medicines are being tested and being released and you may be a candidate for such a product. These medicines either purposefully make you feel nauseated so you won't eat, aid in increasing your activity level so that you burn off more calories, block the fat content of food intake—orlistat (Xenical is the brand name), or like the medicine sibutramine (Meridia is the brand name)—for the reduction of food cravings.

Obesity specialists (bariatrists) also look at obesity as a chronic disease. One of their goals is to have a medication with few if any side effects that can be taken on a daily basis to control and maintain the desired weight. Careful monitoring of blood pressure and pulse rate will be needed with the prescribing of this medication, along with supportive education on exercise and healthful eating. Researchers have still to determine the long-term effects of this medication. Users of this type of medication must be supervised by a health-care professional.

USE OF FOODS

Learning more about foods and their composition may assist in making food choices. If you like a food because of its taste, sometimes it is difficult to eat foods that are less flavorful. Recipes and cookbooks can help. If you are a person who only feels satisfied by a large volume of food, be sure that you drink a glass of water or eat a variety of raw vegetables before sitting down at the table.

The hardest "like" is the use of fats in the diet. Fats do give people the sensation of fullness or satiety faster than any other type of food. Fats also contain the most concentrated source of calories.

Products that contain the new "fat" (olean) may be of assistance, but too much of anything can result in a problem (e.g., diarrhea). Too much of any food—whether it contains carbohydrates, protein, or fat—can lead to an imbalance. Eating the same foods each day will also lead to an imbalance, nutritionally speaking. The goal is to eat a variety of foods over a one- to three-day period in order to obtain adequate vitamins, minerals, fiber, calories, and fluid.

There are a variety of ways to achieve nutritional balance. The exchange system is a method of choosing foods within the six food groups, like vegetables, and getting the number of servings needed for your caloric intake and to meet the needs of your lifestyle and energy expenditure. Counting calories or calorie points has an even greater emphasis on "normal nutrition" (it has to, in order to achieve balanced nutritional results), allowing various choices and combinations of foods.

Combination and amounts of foods (75 calories = 1 point) can also be expanded to the use of carbohydrate (CHO) points (15 gms = 1 point), protein points (7 to 8 gms = 1 point), fat points (2.5 to 5 gms = 1 point), and specific vitamin and mineral points. Carbohydrate counting uses points (15 grams of carbohydrate = 1 point) or just the grams of carbohydrate. If protein is included, a serving of protein is equal to one-half the carbohydrate grams for one serving or one-half a CHO point. Contact the American Diabetes Association for a booklet.

Total Available Glucose is a similar system giving counts of glucose based on the type of food. This program was based on work done by Dr. Alan T. Woodyatt, the physician who also developed the point system.

The American Diabetes Association recommends an evaluation of your present meal plan followed by an assessment related to just making preferably one change at a time. Amounts could be changed. Types of foods could be questioned. The frequency of consuming high-powered drinks or desserts could be altered.

Carbohydrate

Carbohydrate is needed for quick energy and general nutrition. The simple carbohydrate content of fruits and the complex carbohydrate content of grains and vegetables include portions of some of the needed protein and fat content. The variety of fruits and vegetables is even greater in the tropical climates than in the more temperate zones. But with today's marketing, such produce is now available in most areas.

Depending on whether the meal plan is based on high or low carbohydrates (CHO), the percentage of CHO would be one of the earliest considerations. For individual meal plans it would constitute 55 to 65 percent. For other programs 40 percent more or less.

Protein

Protein needs vary with age. The United States, United Kingdom, and Australia include a large use of protein in meals. When protein resources are limited, preference is given to the growing child (15 to 20 percent protein content) and to the older individual (12 to 15 percent is considered adequate). Low-fat proteins are considered the best choices (chicken, fish, nonfat pork chops) for any individual. For an adult, a protein serving the size of a deck of cards is equal to the two to three ounces recommended not more than twice a day. If a person is larger, or if a person is on a low CHO meal plan, larger amounts of protein would be included in the diet plan but not usually over 40 percent.

Fats

Fats become more of a challenge. The use of the limit of 10 percent in saturated fats intake is pretty much in agreement with the American Dietetic Association. The recommended amount of mono- and polyunsaturated fats seems to vary. If you constantly eat less than 20 percent in fat of your total diet, you might not be able to absorb the fat-soluble vitamins such as A, D, E, and K. If you are obese and have Type 2 diabetes, you may have extreme difficulty in losing weight unless you ingest only 10 percent total fat content in your daily intake. Not all health professionals believe this to be true. If including only 10 percent fat in your diet you will need to increase to 20 to 25 percent fat in the diet every four to six weeks so that during this period of time the body will balance out its fat-soluble vitamin needs.

Fiber

High fiber in the diet is recommended but it is not pushed as much by the American Diabetes Association as it was in the 1970s and 1980s. Some of this fiber might be crude fiber (the nonabsorbable kind called insoluble fiber). Dietary fiber (such as found in cereals, called soluble fiber) is found to be more acceptable. Both are helpful. Insoluble fiber is found in whole grain products and corn. It aids in decreasing constipation and colon cancer. Soluble fiber is found mainly in oats, bran, and barley and is an aid in controlling cholesterol levels.

Bulgur, barley, and polenta are useful soluble fibers. They can be cooked in soups and cereals. For insoluble fibers, look to whole grain breads (you actually can see the flakes and seeds in the bread slice) and corn tortillas. These all contain some protein. Another type of protein is available from various beans such as kidney beans (used most often in chili), black beans (especially popular in soups), white beans (also used in chilis), and lentils (an ingredient in minestrone soups).

Vitamins and Minerals

The use of vitamins and minerals becomes an issue when a person diets at a level where the total intake of food does not meet the body's needs for vitamins and minerals. For example, it is said that if you eat fewer than 1,200 calories a day, you will not get all the essential vitamins and minerals because of the lack of volume of food, even if the items consumed represent a balance of types of foods. If calories are restricted in this manner, then the daily use of a multivitamin and mineral tablet is recommended.

Vitamin C is useful for smokers or individuals who are highly stressed (as noted before, purchase vitamin C that includes magnesium and is time released, which is better utilized by the body and results in less impact on the kidneys). Folic acid is recommended as a supplement for women who are pregnant or breast-feeding. Vegetarians may need additional vitamin B_{12}, which is not available through their limited intake of animal products.

Vitamin C concentration has been noted to be lower in people with diabetes. Its use may have some effects on countering cataract development and nerve disorders. Vitamin E has been shown to slow the nonenzymatic protein glycosylation, that is, the connection of glucose to protein (glycated hemoglobin). It is also considered useful in preventing oxidative damage and to reduce the incidence of cataracts.

Vitamin B complex supports energy and endurance. It also has some effect on our emotions and sense of well-being. Stress appears to have an effect on B complex, especially vitamin B_5 (pantothenic acid), which influences the adrenal gland function and vitamin C levels. During high stress times, foods that contain the B and C vitamins or the use of a B complex with C may be helpful. Again, check with your health professional.

B_1 and B_6 may be lower and B_3 elevated in a person with Type 2 diabetes who is experiencing a lot of stress. B_1 is associated with the transmission of nerve impulses and B_6 is associated with motor and sensory activity of certain nerves. Persons with a deficiency of B_{12} may experience a lowering of glycated hemoglobin, indicating an increased erythrocyte or red blood cell population. Niacin (B_3), like zinc, can be dangerous if overused. If ingested in doses higher than 2,000 mg, the result is high blood sugar and liver damage. But in acceptable therapeutic amounts, niacin can lower "bad" LDL cholesterol and triglycerides and raise "good" HDL cholesterol.

If you don't ingest dairy products or have little exposure to the sun, calcium and vitamin D would most likely be needed. Megadoses and/or multiple dose therapy of vitamins have a possibility of being harmful. For example, toxic side effects, such as high blood pressure and kidney damage, are found in individuals who take above 2,000 international units a day of vitamin D for a prolonged period. Another example is that the inappropriate intake of iron may increase the occurrence of atherosclerosis (related to hardening of the arteries).

Calcium is still a must, no matter what its form (vegetables, dairy products), for osteoporosis-prone individuals as well as everyone else; 1,200 grams/day for older individuals and 800 to 1,200 grams for younger to middle-aged individuals are required.

Vitamin E has recently been found to play a role in increasing the immune function, as does the mineral zinc when taken for a short time period (about 2 to 3 weeks). Vitamin E, in 400 to 1,200 international units (IUs), was shown to lower low-density lipoproteins (LDL). One report stated that their subjects experienced a 77 percent drop in the risk of fatal heart attacks that can occur from the blockage of blood to a section of the heart muscle. Note that doses of 1,000 IUs taken for over a year have been associated with depression, excessive bleeding, and the slowing of the time of the healing of cuts and surgical repair. Four hundred IUs is the recommended allowance for adults, according to the latest reports.

Use of antioxidants is being noted more frequently in the diabetes literature. Anitoxidants are vitamins A, C, and E. These substances neutralize free radicals that may contribute to certain diseases like cancer. Studies on the use of these antioxidants have shown that beta-carotene (converted into vitamin A in the body) can be harmful to smokers, making a greater, rather than a lesser risk, for lung cancer.

Manganese may have some role in improving glucose control, but its actual role is still to be determined.

Zinc deficiency only mildly affects glycemic control, but it does appear to be associated with other abnormalities. When zinc was combined with monomethionine, it appeared to have a better ability to get through the acid of the stomach to be absorbed in the small intestine.

Chromium has been associated with a lot of controversy, especially when it comes to diabetes control or prevention, as an aid in weight loss, or for other uses in the body. It does apparently play some role in helping insulin work with glucose. There is no solid proof that chromium is useful above and beyond the very small requirements believed to be needed by the body. It is reported to be easily available from a variety of sources (water, beverages, and in most foods such as meats, dairy products, whole grains, black pepper, and thyme). If the soil in which grains, etc., are grown in is depleted of chromium, then the food made from these grains will not be able to provide chromium to the body.

Chromium is also known to have a tendency to accumulate in the body. A Dartmouth College study found that picolinate, the most frequently used combination in which chromium is found, can damage chromosomes. The body does need the mineral, but there is no solid evidence, at this writing, that it aids in building muscles, lowering cholesterol, or losing weight.

Selenium is also in the limelight. It is found as a part of an enzyme in every cell in the body. Cornell University demonstrated a 17 percent reduction in mortality and a 50 percent reduction in cancer-related deaths among individuals who took 200 mcg of selenium per day, as noted in the vol. 3, no. 10 issue of the *Diabetes Wellness Letter* (call their Helpline: 800-941-4635). It is believed to work with vitamin E to form an antioxidant complex and is found in such foods as chicken, turkey, seafood, and wheat germ.

Vanadyl sulfate (vanadium) is a mineral that has been studied in animals and, more recently, in humans. It is being studied because it is believed to improve the function of insulin. Indirectly, its use by the body is thought to improve glucose tolerance and inhibit cholesterol synthesis. Any supplemental recommendations are premature at this time but seem worth keeping an eye on.

SUMMARY

Which specific vitamin program or plan is best? This is still up for grabs. Proponents for each program say theirs works the best. As reported by a number of descriptive studies, the truth is that less than 40 percent of the population actually follows meal plans. This is the major reason why the ADA recommends what it does. This especially includes restricting the use of concentrated sugars.

OTHER CONSIDERATIONS

Fasting

Fasting is another consideration for losing weight or for those whose religious beliefs promote such practices. Please consult with your physician or other health-care provider before participating in a fast. If you are on insulin, basal insulin requirements need to be calculated. Even if you are not eating, your body still needs insulin to process glucose that is released from the cells. Especially if you have Type 1 diabetes, you may be asked to drink sweetened water so that you will not start burning ketones for energy. If you have Type 1 diabetes, find out what you still need for basal insulin. Often this is one-half of your total daily insulin dosage, proportioned to fit the fasting period.

For any fast, it is also recommended that your fluid level be maintained. Dehydration in the face of the glucose you release from your own cells could result in hyperglycemia without your eating a bite of food.

If you have Type 2 diabetes, guidelines will be determined by the type of oral agent you are taking. If taking an insulin secretory agent, such as repaglinide (Prandin), then you probably will not need to take the medication during that part of the day when you are fasting.

If you are on insulin and an oral agent, reducing the insulin to basal levels may indicate that the oral agent may not be needed.

If you are on an oral agent alone, a hypoglycemic agent may still be needed, but at half the dose. Using other oral agents depends on whether a combination of diabetes medicines is being used and if one or the other combination could be eliminated during that time period of not eating.

Periods of fasting could be for a part of a day, a day, or longer. In most instances, it is recommended that the fast not be more than a day because it could possibly lead to unstable health conditions. For some, this day of fasting may be considered an "internal cleansing" time. Others who fast sunup to sundown, such as for Ramadan, may need to time when the medication could be given, such as after sundown when eating is again permitted.

Recognize that for extended fasts, the third day is the most difficult physiologically. It is not unusual to have nausea or even vomiting on this day. Once these twenty-four to forty-eight hours have been "overcome," a feeling of increased energy usually occurs.

Remember, if you choose to fast, do so with the cooperation of your diabetes heath professional—look at the length of the fast, the type of fast, and the physiological stability of your diabetes management. Return to the usual meal plan, especially after a fast that lasts more than a few days, should be gradual. Eating slowly and distributing foods throughout the day so that the stomach will not suddenly be overloaded will assist the body in readjusting to the food intake.

Glycemic Index

If small amounts of sugar (sucrose, etc.) are included in a food or beverage that is ingested at the middle to end of a meal, it has not been found to cause a great problem in elevating blood glucose levels. That doesn't mean you can put all the sugar you want in that glass of ice tea or eat the full piece of pie, but, in the case of the pie, a few bites at the end of dinner, for most people, won't result in higher blood glucose levels one to two hours later.

The specialists found that the rapidity of absorbtion of foods for one person does not necessarily happen for the next one. Therefore, a glycemic index for you (based on glucose as 100 percent most rapidly absorbed) may be different. An example is ice cream, noted as having a 40 percent glycemic index, but Mr. T. reports blood sugars are in the three hundreds two hours after eating it.

One thing is for sure. Proteins have been found to be more slowly absorbed than fats. If you wish to slow the absorption of food from one meal or snack to the next, include some protein (fats will slow the absorption a little, but again, not as much as a protein-based food). A small amount of disagreement still exists on this and similar subjects. Food labeling is an example of this disagreement.

Food Labeling

You will notice that the percentages on nutritional food labels are based on a 2,000 calorie total daily food intake. But you may only eat 1,200 calories, or perhaps you're very active and you eat 3,500 calories. These percentages do not mean the same to people who are on different caloric intakes. So, is this label information still helpful? It is from the standpoint of stating the total calories per serving size in the particular product, and the percentage of the calories in that product based on fat. The other numbers found below this information may represent more or less than you need.

Carbohydrate (CHO) content is one of these. Although it states the amount in relation to a 2,000-calorie meal plan, it may contain all the CHO you really need to take at one sitting. Same for the fat content.

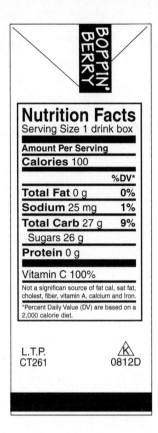

Nutrition Facts
Serving Size 1 drink box

Amount Per Serving
Calories 100

	%DV*
Total Fat 0 g	0%
Sodium 25 mg	1%
Total Carb 27 g	9%
Sugars 26 g	
Protein 0 g	

Vitamin C 100%

Not a significan source of fat cal, sat fat, cholest, fiber, vitamin A, calcium and Iron.

*Percent Daily Value (DV) are based on a 2,000 calorie diet.

L.T.P.
CT261

0812D

Also be aware that on the label are the percentage of Daily Values listings (DV). These listings tell how much of each vitamin and mineral is recommended each day. The DV listing tells what percentage of one serving of that food supplies. If you have questions about this or any of the nutritional supplements, call the American Dietetic Association's consumer line at 800-366-1655.

Watch the ingredients. Note that the largest or most concentrated source of that product is placed first in the list, and then, sequentially, as the percentage of those items found in that product decreases. A good guide to follow is if any form of sugar (dextrose, lactose, glucose, sucrose, corn syrup, etc.) is listed as one of the first three ingredients, it is a product to use sparingly if at all. Also consider limiting or omitting a product if a number of sugars are included later on in the listing. Consider every two sugars to be equal to one step closer "to the top" of the ingredients found in that product.

Soy Products and Green Tea

Soy-based products are useful as part of a meal and especially as a substitute for protein. Four sea vegetables are being used in increasing numbers. The most well known is the wrapping for sushi. This is called nori. Rich in vitamin A, it is usually toasted to a bright green before eating. Another is a variety of kelp: kombu speeds up the cooking time when placed in a pot with beans. It is known for its iodine content and for enhancing the flavor of any other vegetable. Agar-agar is used as a gelatin replacement and is calorie free. Dulse, from the waters of Northern Europe and the northeastern United States, has a light, salty flavor and can be cut up and used in salads, and in place of bacon.

Green tea has been talked about most recently regarding its role in preventing cancer. When the leaves are steamed, rolled, and dried in their processing, it is found that by inactivating enzymes in the leaves oxidation is actually prevented. This does not occur when they are prepared by drying and crushing the leaves. These leaves also contain fluoride and are antioxidant in action.

Green tea is good for the teeth and appears to have an increased potential but not conclusive evidence of antitumor properties. The use of green tea is recommended over the use of other teas for these purposes at this time. (For further information about green tea, call for a copy of the December 1997 issue of the *Berkeley Wellness Letter*: 904-445-6414.)

Supplements are useful when there is a lack of good foods available or when one doesn't choose to eat certain foods considered a part of a healthful meal plan. Vitamin E and other antioxidants have been supported in their use in a variety of ways. Alpha-tocopherol (found in wheat germ and corn oil) is the most common example found on the shelves. Tocotrienol, a vitamin E antioxidant, is a product from rice bran oil. It appears to have an exceptionally good effect on cholesterol levels. If used, its major goal should be to get the low-density lipoproteins below 130 (preferably below 100, especially since you are at high risk having diabetes).

Fluids

Fluid is needed for life. You can only go seventy-two hours without water. It may be obtained by drinking any type of fluid (but pure water is best) or by eating fruits, such as watermelon, that have a high water content. The body needs anywhere from six to ten cups a day. Many drinking glasses hold two cups or sixteen ounces. If you drink this amount at each meal and at bedtime, you easily reach the eight-cup average recommendation.

Water is needed to keep the body temperature regulated and to keep the body chemistry balanced. It also supports chemical metabolic reactions such as those found in the stomach, the intestines, and the blood. Water also assists in the transportation of vitamins and minerals, gases, and waste products.

Most beverages contain 85 percent water and most fruits and vegetables are anywhere from 75 to 90 percent water. Meats, depending on preparation, contain 50 to 70 percent water. Even if you drink only one cup of water per day, you are probably getting anywhere from two to four cups of water from your foods.

Too little or too much water can result in problems. Too much water seldom occurs, but it could be toxic not only from overloading the body with fluid, but also from the minerals and other chemicals found in the water. Elderly people tend to drink too little water. I've heard them say it keeps them from having to go to the bathroom so often. (Note: the base of the Food Guide Pyramid for the elderly is eight cups of water per day.) Too little water leads to anything from heat stroke and heat exhaustion to diabetic ketoacidosis.

Alcohol is a fluid that can enter into the cells without the aid of insulin. It also prevents the release of glucose from your liver, which can lead to hypoglycemia. One or two "dry" drinks (low sugar content, as found in dry wines) per day is the recommended limit.

Drinking alcohol with food, such as during a meal, makes it less of a problem than if it were ingested by itself. To be sure, check your blood glucose levels before and shortly after one drink to learn its effect on you and your blood sugar.

Summary

"Unless you aim for the goal, you can't expect to hit it."
(i.e., normal blood glucose levels) —*Guthrie and Guthrie*

Major health organizations say you can get the nutrients you need through a well-balanced meal plan. By eating whole foods, you may also get some ingredient that, so far, is not contained in pills. An example is phytochemicals, which appear to play a role in good nutrition. Research shows that only a small percent of the population eat well-balanced meals.

All agree that poor nutrition comes about by skipping meals; dieting inappropriately; losing your appetite, especially due to the loss of taste and smell; eating an excess of sugar- and fat-containing foods, or, with older age, not being able to absorb such vitamins as B_6, B_{12}, vitamin D, and calcium. A supplement might be useful if change cannot be brought about by other means.

Remember the adage "If it is too good to be true, it probably is." Stay within the 100 percent RDA dosages unless information is given to support otherwise. Don't be swayed by people's stories. What works for them might not work for you. Studies, so far, have not proven that nutritional supplements can cure arthritis and cancer, but may support the healing or prevention process.

If you decide to use nutritional supplements, choose supplements from companies that have a good reputation. If a product is available by phone or mail, check out the same or similar product in a health food store and then discuss it with your health professional (or use the 800 hotline number of the American Dietetic Association). If an advertisement uses words such as *always, never,* or other *amazing*-type words, do some research before attempting to use such a supplement. When you have the money to buy the foods, or if you eat a balanced meal plan most days and exercise, in most instances you won't need to spend the money on supplements. When special needs arise, with care and caution, certain supplements may be helpful.

Whatever your type of diabetes, recognize that there are key parts of a healthful program that should be part of your program.

- Being active is healthier than being sedentary.
- Take the time to choose wisely the foods you eat.
- Eat only until you feel comfortable.
- Learn the point at which you feel as if you've eaten too much.
- Keep the things that tempt you and are not good for you out of the house, but if you crave a food, take time to eat it infrequently and in small amounts.
- Increase the intensity or duration of exercise when on a weight plateau.
- Build in success for whatever you choose to do. Make changes in small steps.
- Work on positive affirmations so that you feel good about yourself.
- If you start slipping back to habits you don't wish, be aware of them and catch yourself so that you can get back on track.

The conclusion of an article on vitamins and minerals, in the September/October 1992 issue of *The Diabetes Educator,* was if the person with diabetes does not have severe renal function, taking recommended doses of specific vitamins or a multivitamin probably would do no harm and might be beneficial. If you have a complication (such as eye disease, kidney disease, liver disease, or heart disease) and if you have adequate kidney function (especially if fat-soluble vitamins are to be included) taking supplements of certain vitamins such as C and certain minerals, such as magnesium, especially if food intake of these was inadequate, might be helpful. Overall, taking supplements with foods that are natural carriers (taking vitamin C [timed release] with apples and pulped citrus fruits, and carotinoids with green beans, citrus fruits, or broccoli) appears to aid in the absorption.

Dr. Nilsat B. Katz, a physician and biochemist, says at present a case can be made (research supported) for a decrease in calorie and fat intake and an increase for A, E, B_6, folate, calcium, iron, zinc, magnesium, copper, and fiber.

Without careful consideration of meal planning for anyone who has diabetes, the level of blood glucose control cannot be achieved. It does take time and effort, but you're worth it.

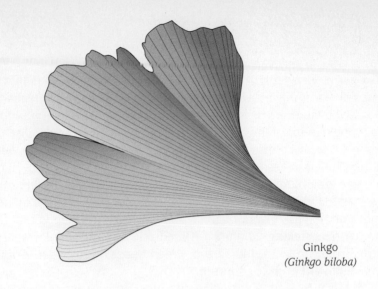

Ginkgo
(*Ginkgo biloba*)

7

HEALING OR HURTING HERBS

Frank was making his first visit to the diabetes specialty clinic where I work. As part of the intake history, I asked if he was taking any vitamins, minerals, herbs, or participating in any therapies. He reported that he had been using a number of herbal remedies. I asked if he remembered the names. When he couldn't, I asked him to bring the bottles to the next clinic visit so that we could talk about what he was taking and how it was helping or hurting him (he did have documented kidney disease).

A week later, he returned clutching his bag of herbal remedies. He was self-administering six different herbs. It was found that two of them could possibly become toxic in the presence of his underactive kidneys. He stated that he noticed that something was bothering him even before this second visit and he had already stopped one of the preparations. Now that he knew he would stop the other.

We discussed the use of the others and the pros and cons for each. I also told him of the various places from which he could get other information on what he was taking. We agreed that if he thought about trying any other herb, he would call or bring that information with him to the clinic. We would study and talk about it with the assistance of the information obtained from the European Commission CD-ROM and the Herbal PDR I keep on hand for such purposes.

THE USE OF HERBS

The use of herbs is more common than most of you might think. Most of the medications taken today originated from some plant first noticed to have healing qualities when used for a certain purpose. There are now so many identified that a CD-ROM disc on herbal remedies would comprise over 4,500 pages of typed words.

These herbal remedies come from all cultures and are used by all races throughout the world. Some herbs are gaining in recognition, while others are a cause for concern, because of toxic effects that result from either mega- or even small dosing. This section is, therefore, only going to include those herbs that may be found to be of greater value to those who have diabetes or those herbs that should be avoided because of side effects and potential toxic properties.

General Considerations

A number of considerations must be weighed before taking herbs. First, the information that follows has been gleaned from a variety of resources, and is to be used for information purposes only. If you find an herb (or vitamin, or mineral) that seems to meet your need, discuss this remedy with a knowledgeable person before using it.

Second, the quality and quantity of these pure products are not regulated by any authority. This means that credibility of the distributor must be ascertained and labels carefully read. Include in this scrutiny an awareness of your own response when taking the herb (or vitamin and mineral) so that you will stop its use with any sign of nausea, headache, or other signs or symptoms that indicate what you have chosen is not right for you. Avoid the use of loose herbs or roots unless you *really* know what you are doing.

Third, be careful about combining any herb with any other herb. There is little information, even though there is scientific study in progress, as to the long-term effects of a number of these herbs, let alone the combined effects when two or more are used at the same time. Make your decisions carefully. Recognize that any problems you might have with kidney or liver function may result from an herb, type of vitamin, or mineral not being adequately eliminated from your body as a waste product.

There was a big uproar when the Food and Drug Administration proposed if any herb, vitamin, or mineral exceeded 150 percent of the RDA, it should be handled like prescription-type drugs. This resulted in the new law, which included all dietary supplements, but still left them less regulated. Through this law, the FDA has to prove danger before pulling a vitamin, a mineral, an herb, an amino acid, and some hormones from the shelves. But there are problems. For example, cholestin could be considered a dietary supplement or a drug, and so it goes on and on.

Availability of Herbs

When you go to a health food store or even to the local supermarket, you will find an overwhelming number of choices of herbs. What should you buy? Is an herb used by the body better when it is taken as a capsule, as a tablet, or as a tincture (often alcohol based)? Do the more expensive products mean that they're better? You might think that because the public is spending more than $3.3 billion a year on these products, something must be working or a lot of people are getting fooled.

Price comparison is useful. Compare for quality, for you can get low-priced herbs that are of high quality and high-priced herbs that are not as sound. Compare among the pharmacy, the grocery store and the health food store, to determine what the best price might be for the same strength of tablet, capsule, or tincture.

If you still have questions when you finish this chapter or at any time, e-mail Prevention@rodalepress.com and ask the "Honest Herbalist" on the subject line. Their resource person, Dr. Varro E. Tyler, is the United States' foremost expert on herbs and plant-derived medicine. As dean emeritus of Purdue University School of Pharmacy and Pharmacal Science, he has authored 270 or more scientific articles and eighteen books.

Europeans have been using herbal remedies more widely over the years. K. H. Waggerl, author of the German book *The Humorous Herbarium,* wrote, "When God, or Lord, made chamomile, he lent it power to ease and heal. That simple flower in patience waits for someone with a stomachache. But pain-racked man, that silly race, puts not faith in commonplace, but calls for pills, says, 'Goodness me! Physician, spare me with your tea!'"

This poem represents the common use of herbs over time when medical men and women were not commonplace. Much of what is found in herbal resource books has been handed down through the centuries. By word of mouth and by written account, each person found out if something worked or not and passed that information on. Of course, the herbs that had minor side effect were probably forgotten and not considered worth remembering, but the others that were poisonous were well remembered.

Safety of Herbs

Some herbs are safe and others are not. A herbal preparation may lead to hypersensitivity. This means you could get anything from a simple rash to anaphylactic shock. This is a serious state that can often be life threatening.

For some preparations, responses are rare. For other preparations, the abnormal responses are more common. There are many people who use royal jelly, and yet it has been repeatedly linked to bronchospasm, a condition in which the bronchial tree of the lungs constricts in spasmlike movements, blocking the passage of air.

Toxicity is another problem. Germander, for example, is a folk remedy used in the United States for its antiseptic properties. In France, it has even been used for weight control. But in 1992 it was reported that there were more than thirty cases of acute liver failure plus one death as a result of the use of this herb. So far, the liver disease was reversed once the herb was stopped. Valerian root, skullcap, and chaparral have all been associated with acute hepatitis or inflammation of the liver. Valerian root, in controlled amounts, is used by Europeans for a variety of problems. Research supports that it binds to brain receptors for mild sedation, leading to improvement of the quality of sleep.

Chinese herbal medicine has also had its problems. The cases are varied, but even with the test of time a toxic response (rash, nausea, or vomiting) can still occur in an individual, and combining Chinese herbal remedies with standard medications has also lead to problems. When they compete for the same pathways in the body, problems can occur.

Other adverse effects have been found in relation to dosage level. Digitalis is an older medication that came from the foxglove plant. It has a very useful effect, but it is carefully given and highly respected for its potential to do harm if the dosage is not correct.

Mahuang is an herb that contains ephedra. Ephedra has stimulant qualities that have resulted in a variety of responses such as creating a rapid and pounding heart rate and raising blood pressure.

Guar gum, used in weight reduction, seemed a simple product, and yet inappropriate use has lead to a death from problems with small bowel and esophageal obstruction.

Contamination is another problem. Without regulation, there may be a variety of contaminants in a product. A kelp (seaweed) product was found to contain small amounts of arsenic (a very strong poison). One herb contaminant was found to be high in lead.

Plants have been accidentally mislabeled, so that a person who thought one herb was being ingested was actually taking a different herb. A number of studies indicated a 4 percent incidence of adverse responses to herbal medications. Another study disclosed that 8 percent of a group of users of herbal medicine experienced side effects.

Regulation Problems

Regulation of these remedies is of concern. People wish to obtain what they want without interference. But the government wants safety to be a priority. With regulation, there is also a concern of higher pricing. Without regulation, there is a concern that more untoward side effects will damage more people. This is a real dilemma.

In contrast, the use of some other herbal remedies elicited fewer side effects than some of the standard drugs. Some other remedies did a better job of improving symptoms than standard remedies. The use of botanical preparations is found in 80 percent of the population worldwide. Although the makers of herbal supplements are not allowed to advertise or state specific health claims, on the label they are able to claim that they assist in improving health. Few people are really conversant with herbs, and directions as to their limited use, such as the anti-inflammatory action of camomile and sabel (sabal serrulata), appear to be free of serious side effects.

In Germany, herbal remedies are registered with the government and guidelines have been established for safe use as 70 percent or more of their doctors use herbal treatments. Commission E is a special group in Germany convened to specifically study and work on the standardization of products. Those products that are available to the public are able to be prescribed by the physician.

In 1994 the Dietary Supplemental Health and Education Act (DSHEA) was passed and signed into law. This law stated that herb products would be listed as dietary supplements. The law allows statements on the labels as to promoting general well-being but prohibits the listing of what the product is used for. The DSHEA also established the Dieting Supplements office, which is a section in the National Institutes of Health. Its function is to collect information and to see that the law is carried out. The key problem is standardization of products so that you get the same percentage of quality herbs in each capsule and liquid or any other form sold.

Usefulness of Herbs

> "Things turn out best for the people who make the best of
> the way things turn out." —*John Wooden*

Ginkgo biloba is being studied for its effect on people who have Alzheimer's disease with its action of increasing blood flow to the brain, improvement of memory, inhibiting platelet clumping, and enhancing the health of blood vessels.

Ginkgo biloba, in its effect on increasing blood flow, reduces cramps in the legs during walking (i.e., intermittent claudication), but clinical trials are needed. Anyone taking an anticoagulant should not confuse the picture by taking this herb, too. More recent research has shown ginkgo playing a role (as does bilberry) to prevent retinopathy.

Saw palmetto has been associated with relieving the discomfort of enlarged prostate glands and acts in decreasing the retention of fluid in the body.

Cranberry for prevention of urinary infections, aloe for wound healing, ginseng as a stimulant, and *Echinacea purpurea* for its antiseptic, antiviral capabilities, are commonly used in this country and are being studied for long-term use and stability in short-term use.*

Echinacea apparently increases the availability of white blood cells in the circulation. Echinacea along with goldenseal is thought to give an added boost to fighting off the symptoms of cold or flu. Concerns

---

*Adapted from "Harmless Herbs? A Review of the Literature," by E. Ernst in *The American Journal of Medicine,* vol. 104(2), pp. 170–178, February 1998.

regarding the use of this herb with Type 1 diabetes will be discussed later in this chapter.

Useful books are Varro Tyler's book, *The Honest Herbal,* and *Herbal Medicines: A Guide for Health Care Professionals,* by Carol Newall. These and many other books promote herbs that are safe and effective. They may also include those herbs suspected of just a placebo effect (i.e., not an actual effect, but a believed effect).

Dangerous Herbs

Dr. Varro E. Tyler, as noted earlier, is a doctor in pharmaceutical science who is well known and respected for his knowledge in the field of herbal medicine (phytomedicinals). Dr. Tyler considers the following herbs dangerous:

- Comfrey used for wound healing is a known carcinogen. Comfrey (and chaparral) can also injure the liver.
- Coltsfoot, used often as a cough suppressant, also has carcinogenic properties along with causing liver and kidney disease and can also injure the liver.
- Germander (or germanium) used for weight loss causes kidney and liver damage.
- Lobelia raises the pulse rate and lowers blood pressure—which could lead to coma.
- Sassafras, as a tonic, is classified as carcinogenic.
- Yohimbe (or yohimbine), used as an aphrodisiac, increases blood pressure and causes a rapid heartbeat. It also may lead to kidney failure.
- Tobacco should also be included on this list. Prolonged use promotes high blood pressure and heart disease. The use of insulin has been found to be less effective in smokers.

Beyond this, there is confusion. Even before this time, when "a wary official" in 1962 refused to approve a sedative called thalidomide, there have been concerns. (When thalidomide was taken during pregnancy, babies were often born without hands or feet.) The law that was passed states that manufacturers could not claim an herb could treat a specific disease. Such labeling is routinely available in other countries.

Another place to check "to be sure" is the American Botanical Council (512-331-8868), where you may place an order for a pamphlet or information about a specific herb.

HERBS ASSOCIATED WITH DIABETES

In the article, "Natural Products and Diabetes Treatment," which appeared in the March/April 1998 issue of *The Diabetes Educator,* herbs were reviewed that have been associated with the treatment of diabetes in some way or another. A key point the authors make is that just because a product is "natural" does not mean it is safe for you to take. They report on a finding that there are some thirty-nine herbal remedies found to make a claim, directly or indirectly, in reference to diabetes treatment. This article also addresses the content and stability of the preparations.

In a magazine called *Phytomedicine,* it was reported that four hundred plants were noted to have glucose-lowering effects. Except for three scientifically based studies, the methodology used to analyzed the plants' effects was weak. It couldn't be stated that 95 percent of the time or greater that the reported hypoglycemic herbs were consistently useful in lowering blood glucose levels directly. (See appendix E for a list of hypo- and hyperglycemic associated herbs.)

The following is a short review of the products people who have diabetes might read or hear about:

- **Akee** fruit does have the ability to lower blood glucose but is too toxic to be used (vomiting and death have occurred).
- **Alfalfa** acts like any fiber plant.
- **Aloe vera** is useful in healing wounds, but it has only a minimal effect on blood sugars when taken internally. Aloe vera has been found mentioned starting about 1500 B.C. and has been used to treat everything from burns and bites, to stomach and intestinal disorders. Today, it is found in shampoos, conditioners, drinks, lotions, and creams. Some products are said to be "better" than others, depending on the type of aloe used.
- **Alpha lipoic acid,** although not an herb, is a potent antioxidant. It also plays a role in balancing glucose. In Europe, alpha lipoic acid has been used for nearly fifty years to treat diabetes and as an antioxidant to treat and prevent polyneuropathy, cataracts, and macular degeneration. A product called "alpha betic" contains the first standardized alpha lipoic acid from Germany's forty years of research. It has demonstrated an ability to promote glucose tolerance, is effective as an antioxidant, and promotes healthy nerve function (800-226-6227).

- **Artichokes** have a very mild effect on blood sugars.
- **Barley** is a fiber but with minimal effect on blood sugars; it does not do as much in controlling blood glucose levels.
- **Bilberry** has been found to aid in preventing retinopathy (diabetes eye disease) through aiding in the blood circulation.
- **Bitter melon** might prove to be useful, if it is offered as a standardized product. In a study it did lower blood sugar 25 percent when ingested over a three-week period.
- **Burdock root** was shown to have some hypoglycemic qualities, but again, no standardization (means you might get a lot in one bottle and little in the next).
- **Capsicum (cayenne pepper)** is being used to treat painful neuropathy in the feet. (Be sure to wash your hands after each application, as the hands can become numb, and if the eyes are touched it can result in extreme pain.) It comes in two strengths. Apply the weakest strength to the feet five to seven times per day for five or more days. If the feet are more comfortable, application is only needed two to three times per day. If the feet are not comfortable enough, repeat this same procedure using the "stronger cream."
- **Chromium** is only useful for chromium-deficient people, as noted by the most current research.
- **Cinnamon** has been known to be useful since 2700 B.C. (in China). It has antiseptic qualities. For diabetes, cinnamon has been shown, by the U.S. Department of Agriculture researchers, to aid insulin and its association in glucose metabolism. For both of these, dosages have not been studied to the point of usefulness in relation to diabetes treatment.
- **CoQ$_{10}$** is also thought to assist the immune system and act as an antioxidant. There is some word on its effect on blood sugars, but as yet there are no strong studies indicating this.
- **Dandelion root** contains inulin (not insulin). It does have a mild effect on lowering blood sugars, but in certain amounts it may be toxic.
- **Echinacea** (the purple **coneflower**), for general use, decreases the symptoms of colds. Don't take it longer than six to eight weeks and carefully consider its use if you are at risk for having Type 1 diabetes. (Use only one-half dose of the tincture for schoolage children and up.) It is not recommended for use in people who have autoimmune diseases (lupus, rheumatoid arthritis, etc.). The logic, not supported scientifically to date, is based on echinacea's impact on a certain part of the immune system. It is believed to enhance the immune

system and possibly also affect the autoimmune system. If the echinacea dose also affects the autoimmune system, then it should not be used by a person that is at high risk of developing Type 1 diabetes. (If you or your health professional are not sure, give yourself the benefit of the doubt and don't use it until more information is available one way or the other.)

- **Ephedra (Mahuang)**—stay away from it. Already damaged blood vessels may be broken with the increase blood pressure associated with this herb.
- **Evening primrose** (contains a linoleic fat) may have a future in treating neuropathy. Evening primrose has been known to ease premenstrual symptoms.
- **Fenugreek seeds** (maple flavor) are high in fiber and have been shown to aid in reducing blood sugar, as noted by studies carried out in India. It is now available under the label of Limitrol. Limitrol is a new way to limit glucose absorption naturally. It also limits fat and calories absorption (800-535-0631).
- **Feverfew,** or **parthenolides,** has been known to prevent migraines, but you have to be taking it a few weeks for it to have an effect on migraine headaches (Canada recently authorized its sale for this purpose). Don't take feverfew when also taking anticoagulants. Pain from a migraine headache can result in elevated blood sugars.
- **Fiber:** juniper, pectin, and glucomanna are high-fiber herbs. Anything that contains psyllium should be high in fiber.
- **Fo-ti** is used by Europeans to treat diabetes, but the research doesn't yet support this treatment as being of significant use.
- **Garlic** thins blood and stimulates the immune system. If you are on aspirin or anticoagulants, check with your health professional, for you may need to alter your dosage amounts. Garlic has been found to have an effect on lowering cholesterol levels but only when the allicin form (pressed garlic) is used. The AGE or aged garlic extract does not show a cholesterol-lowering capacity but does somewhat lower blood glucose levels.
- **Ginger** is said to aid with stomach upset. Some say that it prevents motion sickness when taken one half hour before a trip. Nausea and vomiting could lead to hypoglycemia (low blood sugar). It is possible that eating ginger may result in marked irritation of the stomach.
- **Ginseng** "elevated mood and reduced fasting plasma glucose" when given at certain dosage levels—but it is possible that the increased energy experienced may result in more participation in calorie-burning activities as a result of the elevated mood. Side effects have linked

ginseng to insomnia, diarrhea, vaginal bleeding, and painful breasts. The two-thousand-year-old remedy of ginseng may help relieve stress, as it increases energy and some say it acts as a mild aphrodisiac. It also has been found to affect the immune system. Ginsenosides have been shown to do opposite things, such as raise or lower blood pressure. Those taking ginseng have reported reducing work errors by 31 percent, but it becomes less effective when taken continually. It should not be taken continually more than two to three weeks tops, with a week or so break before restarting.

- **Glucosamine** (doesn't work on glucose) and **chondroitin** are both used by the body to make cartilage. Controlled studies don't give information on long-term use, but sad to say this is true for some allopathic medicines. Their major effect appears to be on easing discomfort, more slowly than standard painkillers but with fewer side effects.

- **Gohsa-jinki-gan** is a combination of ten herbs and appears to be useful in treating diabetic neuropathy. At the 1994 Third International Symposium on Diabetic Neuropathy, Drs. Nishizawa, Sutherland, and Nukada presented information on Kampo medicine. Kampo medicine is the Japanese version of Chinese herbal medicine. This is their traditional medicine, which has been used for 1,500 years. They reported on an animal model of diabetic neuropathy and the use of gosha-jinki-gan or GJK.

- **Grape seed** made into an oil is an antioxidant, but its exact amount of vitamin E is not known. (It is better to get vitamin E in known amounts, in capsules.)

- **Guar gum** is another high-fiber product that is soluble, but it is not readily accepted in its present available forms. It affects blood sugars by slowing down the intestinal action, keeping carbohydrates from being more rapidly absorbed (intestinal blockage possible).

- ***Gymnema sylvestre*** is also known by the Hindi word *gurmar* (meaning "sugar destroying"). The leaves are thought to contain "antidiabetic" properties. It has also been known to deaden the taste bud for sweetness. This herb has been studied in India by the name of GS4. It was found that endogenous insulin secretion was enhanced by gymnema without adverse effects. This is a hypoglycemic that is used in India. It has been demonstrated to help normalize blood glucose levels for people with mild Type 2 diabetes. Toxic side effects have not been noted. It is now available in the United States as Pro-Beta, a proprietary extract derived from the leaves of *Gymnema sylvestre* plant (800-215-3957).

- **Kava kava,** which German research found holds promise for the treatment of anxiety (a person could feel anxious when blood sugars are above or below normal) and topically on teeth and gums for pain relief, has a 20 to 66 percent chance of side effects (nausea, stomach cramps, vomiting) that are reversible once the herb is stopped. Its interactions with other medications or herbs is not known at this time. To date, its use is recommended on a short therapeutic basis (not over four weeks), and not over 300 mg/day.

- **Licorice,** when overeaten, and especially when used by a person with kidney disease (nephropathy), may lead to fluid retention, sodium retention, and hypokalemia (low potassium).

- **Nopal cactua (*Opuntia streptacatha*)** is another plant that is thought to be effective in lowering blood sugar levels. Varro E. Tyler, Ph.D., Sc.D., states that this plant is not available in standardized doses. He states that "using an unstandardized extract of nopal cactus, or any other herb, would be like randomly injecting different quantities of insulin," and therefore, based on present knowledge, it has no place in the treatment of diabetes.

- **Sage,** first noted in Greece to have medicinal value, more recently has been found to have the ability to boost insulin's action. It has also been used as a gargle for a sore throat.

- **St. John's wort** inhibits serotonin reuptake. It should not be taken if you are presently on Prozac, Paxil, or other serotonin reuptake inhibitors. Side effects include fatigue, dizziness, and mild stomach upset. Photosensitivity is possible when using it. It takes four or more weeks to work. Much has been said about St. John's wort (*Hypericum perforatum*) as an antidepressant. It doesn't work as quickly as some of the other antidepressants but appears to be free of serious side effects.

- **Vanadyl sulfate:** it is too early to recommend this for treating diabetes. Research on diabetic rats shows that large doses of vanadium (of which this is a form) may help regulate blood sugar. Limited studies on people with Type 2 diabetes have confirmed some of these results. Not all people with Type 2 diabetes appear to respond to vanadyl sulfate, even in large doses. Large doses have been found to cause cramping and diarrhea. Long-term effects are unknown.

- **Yellow root,** or **goldenseal,** is also used in India to lower blood sugars, perhaps because its bitter taste helps stimulate the loss of appetite. No standardized treatment has yet been proven.

- **Yohimbine** has been used in the treatment of psychologically based erectile dysfunction, but it is one of those herbs that can have dangerous side effects. This must be administered by a qualified person. There are also a number of other herbs that have been used to treat erectile dysfunction, but either they are even less effective or they have greater side effects.

Three other herbs that lower blood sugar are being studied: Madagascar periwinkle, traveler's palm (also known as *Ravenola madagascariensis*—related to the banana plant), and creosote masoprocal (Mother Earth—called "Finger of God" by the early Spanish Settlers; these plants are found in southern France, Italy, and Spain and are described as a leafy stalk with white flowers).

There are now a number of physician's references to botanical medicines that are available through Integrative Medicine Communications (800-217-1938). This information would be useful in increasing the level of knowledge for your family physician of the use of twenty of the most commonly used herbs in the United States.

SPECIALISTS WHO USE HERBS

A number of specialty practices use herbs more readily than the standard physician (unless he or she is a member of the American Association of Holistic Medicine). Naturopaths, homeopaths, chiropractors, practitioners of Ayurvedic medicine and traditional Chinese medicine, and aromatherapists consider the use of herbs in everyday practice.

Naturopaths

Naturopathy or naturopathic medicine is based on the premise that the body has a natural ability to heal. It draws from many cultures, including Ayurvedic medicine, traditional Chinese medicine, Native American medicine, and Hippocratic traditions. The six principles are:

1. the healing power of nature
2. treat the cause rather than the effect
3. first, do no harm
4. treat the whole person
5. the physician is a teacher
6. prevention is the best cure

If you were to go to a naturopathic physician, you would be asked to give a detailed history of your symptoms and complaints, health history, and lifestyle. Then a physical exam and laboratory tests would be performed. The central problem might center on the immune system, or perhaps emotional factors. Then dietary factors would be determined and changes recommended about your general lifestyle. Methods of treatment would be introduced.

The focus in naturopathy is on healing the person rather than the disease. The professionals are trained in clinical nutrition and herbal medicine. They have also been trained in homeopathy, acupuncture, hydrotherapy, physical medicine (which includes micromassage, diathermy, etc.), lifestyle management, and minor surgery (such as sewing up a cut). They are licensed to practice in a few states, and such licensure is increasingly being sought after in other states. There are five major institutes in the United States that train naturopaths. The training lasts four years and longer if specialty training is involved.

Homeopaths

Homeopathic medicine is a nontoxic system of medicine used by persons of other disciplines or by an individual who focuses on just this method of treatment. The name is rooted in the Greek words *homoios* ("similar") and *pathos* ("suffering"). Although homeopathy worries the allopathic physicians in the United States (such as when used in place of traditional allopathic medicine for the treatment for acute pneumonia), the World Health Organization feels that it should be integrated worldwide with conventional medicine.

At present, there are an estimated 3,000 or more medical doctors and other licensed health-care providers practicing homeopathy in the United States. Dr. Hahnemann, who founded homeopathy in the 1800s, based it on the principles of "like cures like," "the more a remedy is diluted, the greater its potency," and "an illness is specific to the individual."

The greater controversy surrounds this diluting principle. Scientists have documented that even if there is only one molecule of a substance in the property, change can occur. The discrepancy comes when some say even without one molecule available, change can take place, as a result of the energy from the original substance being "imprinted" into the homeopathic remedy while it is being diluted. That is, the energy of the original remedy is "absorbed" into the diluting fluid.

If you visit a homeopathic practitioner for a headache, you will find that there are more than two hundred symptom patterns associated with headaches and there is a remedy for each. Details would be asked in relation to position, intensity, position of the body when it occurs, type of person, and other questions to "profile" you as an individual. Your program would be drawn from thousands of tests compiled over two hundred years on healthy individuals and their reactions to sub stances. Other lifestyle alterations would also be considered.

Though there were twenty-two homeopathic teaching institutions in 1900, which almost completely disappeared in the 1930s, homeopathic medicine has now grown into a $150 million industry. Homeopathic medicines or remedies have been accredited by the Food and Drug Administration. A two-hundred-hour course is offered by the British Institute of Homeopathy and College of Homeopathy in Marina Del Ray, California. No state licenses this type of health-care practitioner in the United States.

Chiropractic

Chiropractic practitioners call themselves bone and nerve specialists. They are recognized for their drug-free approach to the treatments of trauma, backaches, and some internal disorders. Their work is based on the spinal alignment of the column acting as a "switchboard" for the nervous system.

Health relies on the balance among the central nervous system (brain and spinal cord), the autonomic nervous system (which controls involuntary functions: heart rate, digestion, glandular function), and the peripheral nervous system (which connects the central nervous system to all body tissues and voluntary muscles). Daniel David Palmer founded the system in 1895 based on early Egyptian practices.

Your visit to this type of practitioner would include your history (family history, dietary history, work history, prior health history), followed by a physical examination. This exam would include a palpation and analysis of the spine to determine imbalances. Very likely an X ray will be taken.

Types of treatment would include an adjustment (the joint is carefully stretched to just beyond its normal range of motion) accompanied by or not accompanied by a popping sound. This is done by hand or by use of a handheld instrument called an activator. Ultrasound or other muscle/nerve stimulating machines might be used for a specified period of time. If you have a fever or other illness, most modern-day chiropractors would attest that their intervention would lead to improved response to the use of allopathic medicine (the standard doctor's regimen), which they would encourage you to seek that very day on completion of their manipulation session.

Most states have a level of licensing for these practitioners, and chiropractors are increasingly covered by more insurance companies.

Training takes four years of undergraduate education (they take the pre-medicine courses) followed by four years in chiropractic education. This may then be followed by other types of specialty training beyond those four years.

Ayurvedic Medicine

Ayurvedic medicine is becoming a more accepted approach to health care, especially based on the work done by Dr. Deepak Chopra. This is a practice that has been in existence for at least five thousand years. Equal emphasis is placed on the body, mind, and spirit. The energy system reference word is *prana.*

The first question the Ayurvedic physician would ask is, "Who is my patient?" The overall health profile or "constitution" of the patient is based on three body types: *vata* (a slender, fast metabolic changeable person—associated with breathing and circulation of the blood); *pitta* (a predictable person of medium build—associated with processing food, air, and water); and *kapha* (the relaxed or heavy body type—associated with bones, muscle, and fat). These body types aid in outlining the program for that person.

On your visit to this practitioner, diagnosis is based on observations, history (past and present—including family), physically examining the body, and listening to the heart, lungs, and intestines. Special attention is paid to the nails, the pulse (six different types of pulses in the right and left wrists), the tongue (discoloration and/or sensitivity), and the eyes. A urine collection would follow: a sweet smell to the urine indicates a diabetic condition and the individual might be asked if "goose bumps" were experienced when passing the urine.

The Ayurvedic doctor would first modify the diet. Protein would be limited, as would fats. Herbal massage and fasting would be the procedure used for Type 2 diabetics only, followed by an herb that is supposed to "cleanse" the liver, pancreas, and spleen. The colon would then be cleansed. These practitioners would be more apt to recommend *Gymnema sylvestre* to stimulate the pancreas and block sugar absorption from the gut; bitter melon for its hypoglycemic effect; and some kind of liver tonic.

Rejuvenation is brought about by the use of special herbs, exercises, or other preparations for the person's specific body type. Then, sound therapy or use of the mind would be prescribed to assist in the healing process. There are presently four schools of training now available in the United States. These schools are there to educate both the public and the professional. No state license is needed (or available) when the person is otherwise credentialed. Practice is to be directly under a qualified health professional trained to interpret this approach.

Traditional Chinese Medicine Physicians

Traditional Chinese medicine combines a variety of modalities. Its history and traditions are over three thousand years old. It has also been selected by the World Health Organization to meet the health-care needs of the twenty-first century.

Traditional Chinese medicine's major focus is prevention, even though there are remedies to treat illness or debilitating conditions. Key parts of this prevention program include education about diet, exercise, rest, relaxation, and stress management. The body is viewed as a reflection of the world. That is why you hear the terms *energy* and *balance* or *yin* (female) and *yang* (male). You can't have one without balancing with the other and maintain health. To keep the *qi* (*chi*) or energy flowing to assist with this balance, certain things must be considered in this five phase theory: Fire (heart—yin, versus small intestine—yang) melts metal (lungs versus large intestine). Metal cuts wood (liver versus gallbladder). Wood penetrates earth (spleen versus stomach), and earth dams water (kidney versus bladder).

On visiting a practitioner of traditional Chinese medicine (TCM), you would first be given an overall inspection. Your body language, tongue, and general appearance would be observed. Then you would be questioned about the symptoms and a history would be taken. While you are talking, the practitioner would be listening to the tone and strength of your voice. He would be attuned to the smell of any body excretions such as the breath or body odor. Palpation or accessing with the fingers the pulse of both wrists, the abdomen, and the meridians (acupuncture points) would lead to the diagnosis. The practitioner would aim to treat the underlying cause as well as the symptoms of the disease.

The traditional Chinese medicine physician would use acupuncture and a combination of herbs. If this is done with a person who has Type 1 diabetes, it must be done early to be effective. The goal for people with Type 2 diabetes is to restore a balance to the endocrine system. Acupuncture has been found helpful in treating neuropathy.

Herbal medicine might be given to you in a paper packet, but more likely in small bottles or containers. The formulas would usually contain more than one substance. In pharmacies in China, these powders would be mixed in response to the "prescription" given by the TCM. Herbs may be boiled in water or taken as a pill, a powder, a syrup, a tincture, inhaled, or as a suppository, an enema, a douche, by soaking, as a plaster, or poultice, or salve.

Acupuncture, cupping, and moxibustion are frequently used. Acupuncture is used to treat the meridian system by directing the response in a specific organ and thereby relieving pain. Cupping is done by heating the air in a flask to cause a vacuum and placing the flask on the affected site. The skin is drawn into the flask by the vacuum and, at the same time, promotes heat to the same area. Moxibustion is used by burning an herb which then smokes. The smoke is guided to the site to be treated.

Massage and manipulation are also used. Massage also promotes and moves energy as it removes blocks or blockages of energy. There are many different types of massage specifically used to meet the need of the seeking person.

Exercise would also be considered as a part of the treatment or recommendation. This would be done on a daily basis such as Tai chi. From the physician's standpoint, the healing type of Tai chi, developed by traditional Chinese healers, would be the use of the therapeutic exercises, one of which is Qigong (*chi-gong*). By means of the focus on the sequence of movements, the person becomes more relaxed, and the internal energy is able to flow without blockages, promoting healing.

Aromatherapist

An aromatherapist is an individual who has been educated, and preferably certified, in the use of the various medicinal properties found in the oils of a variety of plants (termed essential oils). The inhalation (through a diffusor or sprayed into the air or on the skin) from the oils of these plants is only one way to administer treatment, for example, the oil might be given or taken internally (suppositories, capsules, etc.) or be administered by means of massage, bath, or compresses.

The use of aromatherapy dates back thousands of years. Jane Buckle, in her book *Clinical Aromatherapy for Nurses,* reports that lavender (*Lavandula angustifolia*) placed in a carrier oil was used to promote healing through wound cleansing during World War I and was actually approved for such by the French Academy of Medicine. Its ancient history has been noted in such countries as France, the Middle East, China, India, Greece, Europe, and England.

Maurice Gattefosse was first to use the word *aromatherapy* when he discovered, as Ms. Buckle notes, that essential oils take between thirty minutes to twelve hours to be absorbed completely when applied on the skin's surface. She disclosed another study which showed that a number of eucalyptus oils were effective against various viruses including HIV-associated infections.

Oils might be used sequentially to get the combined benefit of each of the individual properties of the specific essential oils, whether they are used in massage or in a compress. An example might be a massage with *Eucalyptus globulus*, which is considered good for arthritis, followed by a ginger-soaked compress (which has analgesic properties). Juniper, an anti-inflammatory, might also be used as a warm soak. Recognize that all of these essential oils are administered in a carrier base.

The chemical makeup of the essential oils contains properties that act as an antibacterial, as a diuretic, as a vasodilator (to enlarge the size of blood vessel openings), as a vasoconstrictor (to decrease the blood vessel tube size), as an antiviral, or as an antispasmodic. Inhaling certain essential oils can decrease congestion of the sinuses. Eucalyptus is probably the most known of the essential oils, as it has been used topically as a chest rub or in a diffusor.

Exacting care must be taken when using a diffusor that contains an essential oil, as lipo-pneumonia (oil inhaled into the lungs) has been documented with "general" use.

A drop of peppermint on the tongue relieves nausea. Tea tree oil may be used for treating wounds, as it has antibacterial and antiviral qualities. *Lavandula angustifolia* is useful in treating insect stings and, when diluted in a carrier oil, for massaging sore muscles/joints (note: there is more that one type of lavender, and each type has specific uses), or promoting relaxation when a few drops are placed in bathwater.

Certain oils must be used with caution, as they are known allergenics. Too much of any type of oil might result in an untoward or abnormal response. Rosemary appears to have a hyperglycemic (high blood sugar) effect. When tested in rabbits previously made diabetic, another study demonstrated that *Eucalyptus citriodora* (lemon-scented gum) had a blood sugar lowering effect (hypoglycemic effect). Education is needed as is research to determine more hyperglycemic and hypoglycemic effects of herbs (see appendix E for lists of hyper- and hypoglycemic herbs).

Nurses may be certified in aromatherapy. Contact the American Holistic Nurses Association for further information (800-278-2462).

Home Remedies

The use of home remedies is becoming more popular because time and money may be saved when home remedies are used carefully and knowledgeably. You can cut off a piece of an aloe plant and hold it on the site, or dab the site with a brown paper bag soaked in white vinegar, or grab an ice cube, to bring relief to minor burns. Washing your feet, two or more times a day, in water that contains one to two capfuls of bleach can keep down and combat fungus of the toenails and skin (e.g., athlete's foot).

Swimmer's ear? A drop or two of a mixture of half vinegar and half water will help. Have an insect bite? Rub full-strength apple cider vinegar on the site. For a sore throat, take one part vinegar to two parts water and gargle. For a room deodorizer, simmer a pan of vinegar and cloves on the stove. Use olive oil not only in cooking but also to soften your skin and to condition your scalp. Olive oil is also useful as a massage oil when combined with a few drops of your favorite perfume. To get the benefits of flaxseed oil, you could buy the capsules or blend two teaspoons with your cottage cheese serving. Flaxseed oil also promotes a shiny coat for animals when small amounts, i.e., a teaspoon, are added to their food. Sesame seed oil rub is considered a useful procedure before or after taking a bath or shower to prevent dry skin.

Chelation

Chelation is a word derived from the Greek, meaning "to claw" or "to bind." Chelation for the specific purpose of decreasing high levels of iron or lead has been successfully used and is considered appropriate therapy for treating lead poisoning in children and adults. Intravenous chelation to remove the plaque from arterial walls is a questionable procedure—especially from a safety standpoint. Chelation removes heavy metals and is considered safe when used in accordance with national protocol.

Chelation by enema can also be problematic because of the fact that electrolytes, vitamins, and minerals might also be removed, along with irritating the intestine, depending on the chelate. Oral chelation, called such when the person uses garlic, vitamin C, zinc, and certain amino acids, is probably safe if megadoses are not prescribed. Observational experiences are reported as positive, but hard, scientific data is either missing or is of concern. It is better not to use this modality unless very sure about the specifics.

There are controversies and there are cautions. Some physicians are trained in the administration of intravenous chelation. Chelation, with its use of a binding chemical in the blood to treat blood vessel disease, must be well understood, and the risks and side effects considered with great care. Other treatments, using chelation, are of more concern.

In 1992, a multicenter study, involving 153 individuals, resulted in nonsignificant differences between those individuals receiving ethyl-enediaminetetraacetic acid (EDTA) as specific chelation intravenously or those who did not, for heart function, kidney function, cholesterol, and triglyceride levels. People were randomized into groups receiving and not receiving EDTA, with the researchers not knowing who was being given what (called a double-blind study). Measurements were taken at the beginning of the study and six months later. Interesting to note, re-searchers found that 60 percent of the control group, or people not re-ceiving the EDTA, reported an improvement in ability to walk a greater distance without difficulty. In a formal review of the literature in 1997, Dr. E. Ernst came to the conclusion that chelation therapy using EDTA for the purpose of reaming out the arteries "should now be considered obsolete"—(or not effective therapy) and should not be used by anyone having diabetes unless absolutely indicated.

You may have difficulty in accepting this, as you may have encoun-tered family members or others who have had positive experiences with the use of this modality. It definitely should not be used during pregnancy, kidney failure, or with a person who has hypoparathy-roidism (which involves low blood circulation). If it didn't have such po-tential for negative side effects, it might be considered one of those modalities that might help but not do any harm. Further information may be obtained by calling 713-583-7666 (the American College of Ad-vancement in Medicine) or 312-266-7246 (American Board of Chelation Therapy).

CONCLUDING THOUGHTS

"The important thing is not to stop questioning."
—*Albert Einstein*

The treatment of diabetes mellitus should balance and stabilize blood glucose levels. Eating properly and getting adequate activity or exercise daily are a must. And even in alternative medicine texts, you would find the usual things like eliminate refined sugars and avoid junk foods. The general meal plan would be skewed toward the high complex carbohy-drate diet with low fat and high fiber.

You might be taught how to test for food intolerances, such as corn, wheat, chocolate, and dairy-related products. Bioflavonoid supple-ments, which have been shown to inhibit the enzyme aldose reductase, and vitamins C, E, and B_6 as well as cod liver oil might each be prescribed, depending on the type of complication present, the prevention desired, or the antioxident intervention sought.

Blood sugars might be used to test individual foods and an "offending" food would be removed from the meal plan. Depending on various needs, B_6, B_2, magnesium, calcium, and antioxidants might be needed as part of the total program. The use of CoQ_{10}, which is thought to aid in stimulating the production of insulin or as an aid in combating cancer, might be included as part of a future program.

A white blood cell or saliva test might let the health professional know if you need zinc. Chromium might be suggested for a person with Type 2 diabetes, especially if it were known that the area's water or soil was chromium deficient. You would be asked to exercise regularly, and to learn some skill, or join some program, or to work within the family to assist in enhancing relaxation practices and for emotional support.

Herbs will not replace insulin therapy where it is needed, especially for a person with Type 1 diabetes. For people with Type 2 diabetes, medication amounts might be lowered or, in some cases, replaced. In general, some herbs that have hypoglycemic or stabilizing qualities might be included to balance out the program. If herbs are used, a close monitoring of blood (for general chemistry, if liver or kidney damage is a possibility, and glucose levels) and urine (for ketones) would be important.

Please note that this chapter and the sections of the appendix that have more information on herbs (C,D,E) do not suggest recommended dosages. The reason is pure and simple. Some dosages are stable and able to be recommended while others are not. Rather than confuse the issue, look them up in the *Physicians' Desk Reference on Herbals* (*Herbal PDR*) and other resources before deciding which dose and for what would be best for you.

Herbal medicine, as a modality, is as old as time. It is making a comeback (in 1998 herb products and related books have reported sales over $5 billion). There is so much that could have been added to this chapter. The information included has only touched on the uses of many herbs and many fields of therapy. An apology is made if I didn't include your area of interest, or include other modalities that might be of less interest, but of more concern. You should have, at least, found out something you didn't know before. I hope, you will be challenged to learn more.

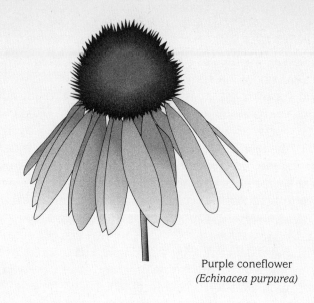

Purple coneflower
(Echinacea purpurea)

8

SIGHT, SOUND, AND SELF-MANAGEMENT

Annette accompanied her mother on her clinic visit concerning her mother's poor Type 2 blood sugar control. The blood glucose levels were responding to treatment by becoming lower and more stable, but only when her mother took her medicine. Her mother was increasingly becoming more depressed.

The daughter said, out of earshot from her mother, "I don't know what to do. My mother says she doesn't care anymore about anything and has even refused the antidepressant medication her family physician prescribed. She said she just didn't want to take another pill."

I asked her if she had ever listened to music therapeutically. Then I asked about the types of music her mother liked when she told me that she didn't know there was such a thing as therapeutic music. We talked about using brighter music in the morning and during the day and a quieter type of music during the evening.

A week later, I received a phone call from Annette. She wondered why someone had not told her about the use of music before. Her mother was much brighter and she was now taking her diabetes medication. Most of her blood sugars were now normal.

THE POWER OF ENERGY

"Wisdom begins in wonder." —Socrates

This is one of the most complex and yet the most helpful chapters of the book. You had the opportunity in chapter 2 to read about mind/body function and tools for creating positive thinking. Assertiveness covers a variety of modalities that more often than not are not considered alternative or complementary, since they have been previously recognized as coping mechanisms. Relaxation includes ways to reach a state of calm and peaceful thinking or mindfulness meditation through various relaxation practices. Exercise includes other mind/body activities. Chapter 6, on nutrition, includes antioxidant and vitamin and mineral information, and chapter 7 included some of the most recent herbal information and aromatherapy.

What is left are the fields of manual healing (part of which could be considered under Relaxation) and bioelectromagnetic applications. The first of these two sections (chapter 8) will focus on those therapies that affect sight and sound, and those therapies that guide self-management (to give you a different view of how important your self-care techniques may be) after a review of energy therapy, which was initially addressed in chapter 1. The second section will cover techniques and therapeutic use of touch and nontouch methodologies (chapter 9).

ENERGY MEDICINE

People probably don't think about energy medicine, but they will increasingly read and hear this term used. The educated few are probably thinking about therapeutic touch (TT), or Reiki, or healing touch (HT). Energy medicine is really a broad umbrella that includes everything from what you feel, see, touch, smell, sense, taste, and experience. Heat is energy. Cold is energy. The state of being calm is a different type of energy, as is the aroma from cooking foods. As was noted before, energy is a life force. So, whatever name it is given in whatever language, it represents a change in dimension and movement that is occurring all the time.

It is stated that everything is made of moving particles, some more dense than others (i.e., like a "solid" piece of furniture). Just as resistance is felt when you try to put the two positive ends of a magnet together, so is energy used in our everyday life in keeping healthy: putting cold water on a burned area of the skin; using vaporizers to assist in breathing when nasal congestion occurs, etc.

Energy Names

Here are some names that energy is given (it seems as if various cultures recognized energy in various forms and therefore needed to name this *vital energy*): Hebrews called it *ruach*. The Japanese used the term *ki*. India named it *prana*. Egyptians called it *ankh*. China uses the term *qi*, or more popularly known as *chi*. Tibetan medicine people call this energy *lung*, with the *u* pronounced *oo*.

In energy medicine these networks or energy channels are seen as "vessels" that pipe energy from a coordinating center. These centers are called chakras. Chakras represent different functioning of the body and are noted by various colors similar in sequence to rainbow colors, and by various tones, by various symbols, by various gemstones, and by various responses to a pendulum held above the center of the specific chakra or energy center and others that will not be discussed in this book.

The root chakra is red, and associated with physical well-being. The second chakra is represented by the color orange and is associated with reproduction. The solar plexis chakra is yellow and associated with digestion and the autonomic nervous system. The heart chakra (gold or pink) represents the center and circulatory activity. The throat chakra is fifth (light blue). The "third eye" or point of wisdom (found on the forehead) is represented by violet and interacts with the head (not including the brain) and central nervous system. The seventh or crown chakra is white and represents or centers the action of the cerebrum (major part of the brain).

Psychoneuroimmunology

As the field of psychoneuroimmunology (the study of the interaction of the mind, nerves, and the immune system) maps out its knowledge of the body's energy capabilities. It has been able to recognize the associations of the various energy centers of the body and the interaction of hormones or chemicals called neuropolypeptides that are secreted throughout the body and have receptors in other parts of the body. This helps you understand why when you are depressed, you are depressed all over. When you feel pain, you experience that pain in a generalized way. With referred pain (pain that is felt other than at the site of injury or infection), or ghost pain (pain that is felt in a part of the body that has been amputated), the site of the pain is different from the source of the pain.

The power of energy manipulation could be everything from a Buddhist monk altering his internal temperature so that he experienced no cold or frostbite from standing in snow, barefooted, in 20 degree Fahrenheit weather, to walking into a rest room in a modern building and having the light turn on without your having to touch the light switch.

All of this is from quantum physics, which is based on Einstein's theory of relativity. His theory is that all matter is energy in motion (like the molecules in the light switch just recently mentioned). Alternatively, Newtonian physics considers one response as simply the result of another response—the philosophy behind conventional medicine.

THERAPIES

"The best and most beautiful things in the world cannot be seen or even touched. They must be felt with the heart."
—Helen Keller

The therapies and actions discussed in this section have something to do, directly or indirectly, with various energy responses of the mind/body. (Chapter 9 discusses the techniques and therapies that you, more often than not, may associate with energy therapy.) Those that are covered in this chapter are associated less with energy medicine, but from the implications themselves, they are energy-based modalities. Even the simple form of art therapy is an expression, as exercise is movement, and a response to mental, physical, emotional, and spiritual stimuli.

Art Therapy

The use of drawings as art therapy is not one of the modalities found in standard alternative and complementary texts, and yet it is a useful tool to find out where you are and what changes you have made. Drawing a picture just for yourself is really nonthreatening, especially if you feel you don't have to show the drawing to anyone else. Yes, there are books and manuals to interpret drawings for things like impulsivity, anger, insecurity, or other emotional qualities—but for you, doing a drawing just becomes an outlet and a release instead of having to take a pill.

If you are under treatment for any chronic illness, a drawing can express how you feel about that illness. An example of this is the ten-year-old child who drew her interpretation of "diabetes." Her picture was painted solid black except for a little corner of the picture that held the word *diabetes*. The family who felt their daughter had to get used to the outside world chose not to change their self-care and eating habits and therefore refused to go or have their child go to counseling. The outcome was disaster. Six years later the suicide note she left said "why should I take care of myself when my family doesn't take care of themselves?"

Another example of the usefulness of art therapy is the woman who drew nothing but a big *D* when she was first diagnosed with diabetes. As she became more adjusted to having diabetes mellitus, she found herself drawing smaller and smaller *D*s until finally the *D* actually became a flower. Therefore, a drawing may give you psychological insight into your true feelings about what is happening at the time.

Take a moment to draw your interpretation of what diabetes means to you. Are you using heavy strokes and dark colors? Do you find yourself focusing on your place in the family since you've had diabetes, as is seen by your placement in the picture in relation to the rest of the family members? How are you seeing yourself experiencing an insulin reaction (low blood sugar) or using syringes or blood glucose monitoring devices? Just as there are books on the interpretations of dreams, so there are books on the interpretations of drawings.

A word of caution. You should not overly interpret what the drawing means, but it can give some insight into more deep-seated emotional problems than you might be unable to put into words. This would be only one piece of information that might result in a need for further assistance.

Aromatherapy

Aromatherapy has been discussed, in part, under the listings found in the chapter 7. But here it is discussed from a different basis. A few drops of an essential oil such as coriander can be placed in a carrier base, like olive oil, or grape seed oil, or almond oil, or canola oil, and massaged into a muscle to relieve pain and muscle spasms. Sandalwood has also been known for ages to relieve muscle spasms. A carrier base could also be a tub of bathwater or any container of heated water.

Whether they are used directly or indirectly in some carrier base, the essential oil may come from any part of the plant. Note that an essential oil coming from one part of the plant might be helpful whereas one coming from another part of the plant might be irritating or harmful.

Tea tree increases immunity and fights infections along with its ability to bring about a calm feeling during emotional stress. The odor of this essential oil can trigger various responses in the body, from memory association to actual physical responses. It is also known to stimulate the release of neurotransmitters and endorphins (which can give you a sense of well-being) in the brain. Recently, tea tree oil was reported, from a scientifically based study, to treat fungal infection of the toenails at the same rate as a prescribed medicine (takes eight to ten months or more).

As with any other therapy, safety is a factor. If used on the skin, watch for any signs of allergic response. In fact, it is not a bad idea to put a drop of the diluted essential oil (the oil in the carrier base) on the area of the body to be massaged. Then, wait a short time to see if any irritation becomes apparent before massaging it into the skin. The scent of the oil in combination with the massage leads, as you might expect, to muscle relaxation. But if the scent bothers the individual, then even the massage with that oil might not fulfill the purpose for which it was intended. Courses are offered for further education in this field as well as many other fields (800-877-1600).

Colon Therapy

Colon therapy could be considered a form of chelation therapy, as it alters the electrolyte or chemical balance of the body in some way. Perhaps this is a good time to mention that anything that changes the chemical balance of the body is more serious for someone who has diabetes.

From the time of the early Egyptians and Greeks, physicians have administered colon therapy or enemas as internal body baths. It was introduced to the United States in the 1890s; Dr. John Harvey Kellogg used colon therapy to avoid doing surgery on his patients who had gastrointestinal disease.

Colon therapy was also used to treat high blood pressure, infections, heart disease, arthritis, and even depression, as noted in the book *The*

Alternative Medicine Handbook by Barrie Cassileth, Ph.D. After antibiotics became availabe, the major use of colon therapy became "detoxification." Although most of this is done by enema, colon cleansing is also carried out by laxative-type substances or herbs administered by mouth.

Research is concerned about this practice, which is based on the assumption that "mucoid-forming foods" remain in the colon, and this gluelike substance needs to be removed. But when medical doctors have scoped the colon to examine the intestine for bowel cancer over the last twenty years or so, no such coating or sticky residue was found. With the resurgence of the use of this therapy in the 1990s, deaths did occur, but they were more often the result of unsterile conditions or the type of herb or other substance being placed in the fluid before being given in an enema.

This therapy is never to be used for anyone with intestinal disease or tumors. Even the colon therapists recognize this caution. Enemas to relieve constipation or for diagnostic purposes, like a barium enema, are considered acceptable. A session may last from thirty to forty-five minutes and uses an average of four quarts of water.

The more potentially health-threatening "high colonics" are meant to clean out the entire colon. The president of the American Colon Therapy Association states that such therapy can help alleviate bad breath, gas and bloating, tiredness, and sinus or lung congestion. Again, if diabetic diarrhea is present, that is considered an intestinal disease, and the pooling of fluid in the intestine and the overabsorption of such fluid could lead to water toxicity or other problems, depending on what the fluid contains. Further information may be obtained from the American Colon Therapy Association (210-366-2888) or the Gastro-Intestinal Research Foundation in Chicago (312-332-1350).

An alternative to remember is that if whole foods are eaten that contain high fiber and adequate nutrients, constipation is less apt to occur. Unless you have gastroparesis or diabetic diarrhea—the second of which is recognizable when part of the intestine lacks the nerves to support peristalsis or the usual fifteen contractive movements per minute—normal functioning would be expected in most adults and compromised in older adults only if the fiber and fluid intake are less than desired.

Chiropractic Therapy

Chiropractic (from a Greek word meaning "done by hand") care (formerly discussed as a field that may recommend herbal therapy) is a growing occupation in the United States. An increasing number of states are licensing this practice and a greater number of insurance companies are covering some of the cost of its use. This modality is based on the concept of the body's ability to heal itself during times of physical injury or mental and environmental stress. This is done through "adjustments" of the spine and joints, which, in turn, influence the nervous system and associated defense mechanisms of the body.

Chiropody was introduced in 1895 by Daniel David Palmer, who was a student of physiology and anatomy. Although he was the first to formalize training in this field, apparently spinal adjustment has been around since early Egyptian and Greek (Hippocrates—fifth century B.C.) times. Dr. Eisenberg, in the 1990s, found that 10 percent of the population used chiropractic.

These health-care providers look at the spine as the "switchboard" of the body. When you visit them, they take a history, which includes everything from dietary habits to where and how you work. The physical exam includes a thorough evaluation of your spine and is often followed by one or more X rays. Chiropractors are looking for displaced or dislocated vertebrae that block the energy flow—called subluxation. The quick thrusts or adjustments to the spine are thought to correct this problem. They have a strong belief that disorders of the spine relate to or are the underlying factors of disease.

The chiropractor has a variety of therapies to offer. It is possible that a patient may be referred to an internist, pediatrician, or neurologist for further studies.

In the case of illness, the chiropractor would align the spine so that the individual would respond better to the treatment of the allopathic physician (your family doctor). A resource for further information is the American Chiropractic Association (703-276-8899). Problems appear to arise most often when the chiropractor goes out of the sphere of training or when he or she uses the premise that spinal manipulation can cure internal disease. Otherwise, it has been considered useful for relieving acute low back pain, neck pain, and possibly for headaches that do not seem to respond to other therapy. A 1992 report (Rand Corporation study) concluded that manipulation for low back pain is more effective, safer, and less expensive than traditional medical care.

Osteopathic Therapy

Osteopathy actually started a few years before chiropractic therapy. It was developed and promoted by Dr. Andrew Taylor Still in 1892 in a town about a day's journey from Mr. Palmer's. While chiropractors generally focus on the spine, osteopathy uses arms and legs as turning points for bending and twisting the body.

Osteopathic physicians learn both conventional medicine as well as their rotating or fulcrum manipulative techniques. Many osteopaths do not use manipulation in their practice. In fact, going to an osteopath might seem the same as going to a standard allopathic doctor, but more and more osteopaths are using manipulation and assessment practices taught as part of their basic education program.

Osteopaths take the same state board of examinations as traditional physicians (allopathic). There are four years of osteopathic school followed by one year of internship and possible specialty training beyond that, often completed in an allopathic setting.

Homeopathic Therapy

Homeopathy was first discussed in chapter 7, on herbs. It's another field that has considerable controversy associated with it. Once there were twenty-two schools teaching homeopathy in the United States. Now there is only one, as noted previously.

Samuel Hahnemann, a German physician, around the turn of the nineteenth century, invented homeopathy. It actually dates back to the writings of Hippocrates, who noted that disease is cured through "application of the like." Hindu physicians described what is still known as the Law of Similars. Dr. Hahnemann's approach was based on three principles:

- The first principle is the Law of Similars or "like cures like." This is explained that a substance that causes certain symptoms can cure a person suffering from those same symptoms, if taken in small doses (similar to the philosophy behind vaccinations).
- The second principle is the Law of Infinitesimals. This means that the more dilute the dose, the more powerful its effect.
- The third principle is the Law of Chronic Disease. This principle states that treatment with medicine, whether herbs or drugs—which Dr. Hahnemann called "allopathic"—drives the illness deeper into the body, while his remedies release the problem and produce "true healing from within."

The Law of Proving suggests criteria for evaluating the effect of substances on the healing responses. Dr. Hahnemann and his assistants actually ingested plants and other substances to record the symptoms each substance produced. They were then treated with diluted doses of the substance.

The father of American homeopathy in the mid-nineteenth century, was Dr. Constantine Hering. Hering's Law of Cure states that the healing that occurs progresses from the deepest part of the body to the extremities. Thus homeopaths believe they can track the progress of healing "layer by layer."

If you go to a person who practices classical homeopathy, the doctor would take a full assessment of your symptoms and personality characteristics. Then, the practicing homeopathy physician would determine a substance that produces a similar effect when taken in toxic doses. This would be done by referring to the *Homeopathic Pharmacopoeia of the United States* (first published in 1897). This health provider would then prescribe this remedy in a special diluted preparation. Interestingly, it is believed that the greater the dilution the stronger the potency, due to the energy transferred to the diluent.

If the dilution is shaken between each subsequent dilution, it is believed that the energy of the molecules are transmitted to the diluent or fluid used for diluting the dose. Even when there is not a molecule of the original dose left (noted after a thirty times dilution factor), there is still believed to be an "imprinting" of the original dose on the diluent.

The "imprinting" factor is yet to be proven. Still, people have found relief, placebo effect or not, with the use of these products. Needless to say, they are not harmful, and they are regulated by the Food and Drug Administration.

Classical homeopathy is a very holistic therapy. The simplified form focuses on a particular disease or symptom and could be called symptomatic homeopathy. This is an approach to care that is largely practiced by naturopaths, who may prescribe both herbs and homeopathic remedies.

Since side effects are not a problem in the use of homeopathy preparations, for common ailments (cold, allergies, stomach upset), use would most likely not be reflected in changes of blood sugars other than those associated with healing (the body returns to the previous level of blood sugar control). Be sure to contact your health professional if blood sugars are not responding to any change in diabetes treatment (such as blood sugar to more than 250) and moderate to large amounts of ketones are present in the urine four to six hours after intervening with recommended, traditional therapy.

Other information may be obtained from the Homeopathic Educational Services (800-359-9051) and the British Institute of Homeopathy and College of Homeopathy (310-306-5408).

Hypnotherapy

Clinical hypnotherapy is useful in a variety of settings. Hypnotherapy may be used for psychotherapy, but the type discussed here is that which is self-induced and self-managed. This can be particularly helpful, no matter what the focus, in calming you, and calming yourself results in lower blood glucose levels.

Dr. Milton Erickson, a famous psychiatrist and hypnotist, said that there was no such thing as a nonhypnotizable person. For Ericksonians, a daydream, or being focused on the lines of the highway, are types of hypnosis. So, no matter if you think you are not hypnotizable, think about that book that you couldn't put down, and while reading it you were not aware of others in the room. In other words, you are just more or less easily able to get into this state of deep concentration. You are in control at all times unless suggestions are given in a way that the person accepts as reasonable and, in reality, they are not. An example would be the person who uses a real gun with the mistaken belief it is a water gun.

Training allows people to place themselves in a state in which they are alert and yet relaxed and capable of feeling less uncomfortable or less anxious by learning to concentrate on what is most appropriate for them. Through this therapy, blood glucose levels may be increased or decreased, skin temperature changed, and gastrointestinal activity altered.

The relaxing component of hypnosis should promote the lowering of blood glucose levels (as would any relaxation therapy). The word *hypnos,* based on the Greek word meaning "to sleep," is really not associated with a sleep state or delta rhythm. It is usually associated with the theta rhythm measured at four to seven cycles per second. Or when the person is in a "lighter state" (alpha state), which records the brain's waves at thirteen to thirty cycles per second. Both of these states may be experienced in the awake state.

Mesmer, a German physician, was the first to use such an intervention and was actually banned from France when the medical establishment could not verify his work. Others, such as the English surgeon James Esdaile and Sigmund Freud, used hypnosis, even though Freud later discredited it. Surgery has been performed while the patient was in a hypnotized state. Dental procedures have become more bearable while the person's under hypnosis.

Again, the patient is always in control and can alter his/her state of consciousness to a more alert state at any time. The therapist is only the guide for the process. The use of this therapy in quitting smoking, controlling or suppression of appetite, controlling fears or phobias, and altering painful states has been of help to many people. Solid research now documents the response of the brain waves in both adults and children. It is not meant to cure anything, but basically it allows you to be in a state in which there is a focus on change or control of physiological functioning. The American Institute of Hypnotherapy (714-261-6400) and the American Society of Clinical Hypnosis (708-297-3317) can send you information on the use and safety of this modality.

Again, if you were having a hypnotherapy experience with a certified hypnotherapist, you would find yourself in a pleasant room, and with the Ericksonian approach rather than the traditional approach to hypnotherapy (more autocratic), you would be asked to breathe comfortably and either keep your eyes opened or closed. If you felt your eyelids getting heavier and heavier, you could close your eyes and thereby relax the muscles around the eyes and also block being distracted by what you see. You might be asked to include or allow the sounds in the environment to aid or signal you into becoming more relaxed. You might be asked to raise your arm if it feels light to you or to move a finger when you feel you are the most relaxed.

Suggestions might be given as to what to remember, or to do after the session, recognizing that you could, if you choose, remember anything you wished to at any time. The hypnotist might find out before the session or during the session if you felt more relaxed going up or going down; feeling heavier or feeling lighter; using the visualization of an escalator or a flight of stairs. When it was time to end the session, you would be guided to become more alert. If you liked the relaxed state you were in, you might decide you didn't want to be more alert at that time so you could choose not to be more alert. When you were ready, you could open your eyes and then share your experience with the therapist as much or as little as you wished. If you were concerned about any feelings you had either during or after the session, you could disclose the information, block the information, or forget the information, as you wished.

Although hypnosis is safe for self-practice and for therapy, caution should be used when treating people who are psychotic or have antisocial personality disorders. This is a directive from the World Health Organization.

Imagery Therapy

As with the possibility of any hypnotic state, imagery can directly affect a person's physiology. It can affect damaged cells and increase or decrease circulation to a damaged site just through the active power of the mind. The radiation cancer specialist Dr. O. Carl Simonton performed research in the use of imagery for people with cancer and demonstrated a higher degree of healing, a feeling of greater self-control, and increase of self-esteem with the use of guided imagery.

Researchers have found the Positive Emission Tomagraphy (PET) scan to be most useful in examining brain tissue. Through the use of a type of glucose injected in the bloodstream, PET can show which parts of the brain are active when a person visualizes something (such as a part of the brain that uses up the glucose quicker). Notable changes have been seen in response to various emotions aroused by the use of guided imagery. Guided imagery can be useful in pain control, gaining insight into feelings, increasing self-esteem and physical healing.

Dr. Martin Rossman is the cofounder of the Academy for Guided Imagery (800-726-2070).

The following is a guided imagery exercise that you may tape and use when needed. Close your eyes, if you wish:

Imagine yourself climbing a mountain, the mountain representing the problems associated with having diabetes. . . . As you climb, you find yourself up against a cliff and you seem to be blocked from going any higher. . . . Just then, a hand reaches down to assist you over what seems to be a section of the way that is impossible to overcome. . . . You are lifted on to the higher path. You continue to proceed upward, encountering various problems as you go on. . . . Finally, you reach the top of the mountain. How beautiful and peaceful it is . . . Be by yourself or have others join you. . . . Notice the freedom and openness you feel. . . . As you look out, you see other mountains and come to the realization that since you have reached the top of this mountain you know you will be able to reach the top of many other mountains to come. . . . Sense the joy in being able to accomplish such a task as this. . . . When you are ready, open your eyes and write down your thoughts.

Journaling Therapy

Keep a pad or notebook handy. Placing writing materials at the bedside is useful, especially for those nights when you awaken with many thoughts that keep you from going to sleep. You will note that once those thoughts are transferred to paper, then it is much easier to return to a state of restfulness. Write short notes or long paragraphs. This is just for you, so the handwriting doesn't need to be neat (just legible enough so that you can read it at a later date, if you so choose).

Hug Therapy

For the fun of it and actually for its therapeutic value, consider hug therapy. Hugging or embracing comes from the Scandinavian word, *hugga,* meaning "to soothe or console." It raises the pulse rate, and thereby increases the circulation. It often puts a smile on a face or consoles a tearful person. I'd even bet the immune system benefits when one is hugged. Most likely the blood sugar would go up somewhat for a short time with the surge of adrenaline that is released into the bloodstream.

The most famous hug of all is the bear hug. This is done gently, but firmly. If the legs as well as the arms are involved, then this hug can be thought of as an "octopus hug."

An A-frame hug is done when just the upper part of the body is involved in the hug. A buddy hug is done by putting your arm around someone's shoulder and giving a squeeze. An arm hug is usually done around the waist of the other person, or it could just be done by squeezing an arm.

Little people give knee hugs. Big people give hand hugs. A two-handed hand hug is more meaningful than a one-handed hand hug. The sandwich hug is known for incorporating more than two people. If it's a prolonged hug, it is often considered a snuggle.

There is hug etiquette. Unless you know the person really well, always ask before giving a hug. Some people, because of unfortunate experiences in their lives, have difficulty being hugged—and would rather not hug. Then there is the truism that the more hugs you give, the more hugs you get.

There is the prescription that four hugs a day is mandatory—meaning that they are really needed to function properly. If you are ill or things are not going well, then the prescription is twelve hugs a day. Twelve hugs a day is considered therapeutic, as June Bierman and Barbara Toohey say (authors of such books as *The Peripatetic Diabetic,* and *The Diabetic's Total Health Book.* Their website is www.diabeteswebsite.com).

Music Therapy

Music therapy is also of use, especially when no one else is around. It is also useful for groups as well as individuals. It can brighten spirits or calm them down, depending on the type of music played. You've heard of "elevator music"? It is as it sounds: during the early part of the day, the music is brighter and more energetic—urging you into being awake and doing a lot of work. Toward the end of the workday, the music becomes more calming—soothing ruffled feelings and bringing to close the day's activities.

Music is powerful. Remember, discordant music can shrivel cells, while pleasant music can promote cell growth. A good resource is the noted music therapist Janalea Hoffman, who may be reached through the order line of 888-JANALEA.

Music that is paced at fifty beats per minutes is calming and relaxing. It can also provide a quiet background for study.

Music energizes the body through vibration: place your hand on your cheek as you hum a tune. Singing or humming is stress relieving. If you are in heavy traffic, sing a song. Don Campbell, an educator specializing in sound, suggests using music for relaxation, meditation, and invigoration, as well as using music for going to work, music to enhance concentration, music to get up to, and music to go to sleep by, music for inspiration, and music to stimulate imagery.

Music has assisted in healing. Music sets the stage for the body to be in balance and thereby supports the healing process. In the July/August 1998 issue of *Complementary Medicine for the Physician,* Michael Thaut, Ph.D., wrote "Music therapy: the unsung modality." He notes that music is the result of personal preferences that have been noted in various cultures around the world and throughout time. Music stimulates memories and results in physical movement "as the beat goes on."

Music therapy is so called when music is used to achieve therapeutic goals. Music could be used to increase exercise compliance. Learning to play an instrument helps a child or an adult to enhance their ability to focus. Music soothes those who are agitated (depending on the choice of music).

Other research into the use of music has shown it can effect changes in emotional responses. Fewer errors were noted when a certain type of music was played. Music has been shown to lower heart rate and blood pressure. Music has also found its place in neurological rehabilitation. Singing shifts the brain dominance from the critical left to the creative right.

Further research has shown that sound puts the motor system in a state of alertness. People move more quickly when listening to lively music. Marching band music may not only stimulate memories of another time, but can also pick up the heart rate.

Music therapy is used to decrease pain, to calm an individual, or to get a person moving. If you are a person who has trouble sleeping, playing quiet music can aid the body in being more receptive to rest. If your neighborhood is too dangerous for you to go walking, get out the music and dance.

If you want some further guidance, call 301-589-3300 to obtain the name of the closest board-certified music therapist in your area (from the American Music Therapy Association). Check out their web site at www.musictherapy.org.

Magnet Therapy

Magnet therapy is another form of touch but with a slightly different focus. You may know someone who wears magnetic insoles, or wrist or back wraps, or who sleeps on a magnetic pad. Often they will state that what pain they experienced had been lessened. You wonder if this is for real. Also, how does it work?

How magnets actually work is not known, but it has been theorized that such devices increase blood flow to the affected area and directly or indirectly work on neurotransmitters that are associated with pain messages. They perhaps create a small electrical current that blocks, somewhat, the sensation of pain.

Still another source theorizes that magnets improve the ability of red blood cells to carry oxygen. Scientific studies about magnets are now in progress. Clinical studies have shown about an average of 50 percent positive responses. Magnets are not believed to heal anything but only to facilitate the healing process.

When the astronauts first returned from space, they couldn't understand why it took six weeks for them to recuperate. When researchers recognized that the astronauts were outside the magnetic field of the earth, they added magnetic material to their suits. They no longer have this lag time in returning to earth.

There is a question as to whether magnets are safe over the long term, short term, or both, and yet MRI, or magnetic resonance imaging, is replacing X rays because of the safety and accuracy factor, and magnetoencephalography is now replacing electroencephalography for recording brain activity. More research needs to be done, because exposure to electromagnetic fields has been correlated with reports of depression, suicides, chromosomal abnormalities, learning difficulties, miscarriages, and brain tumors compared to the unexposed groups.

Magnets are expensive. Not all are the same. Permanent magnets are similar to refrigerator magnets. These might be sewn into wraps or used as magnetic strips. Pulsed electromagnetic field magnets are coils wrapped with copper wire that have an electrical source such as a battery or wall outlet. This device generates the magnetic field by passing current through the coils. The permanent magnets appear to improve blood flow, while the pulsed electromagnets work on changes at the cellular level.

In Germany, the use of magnetic devices is covered by medical insurance. Treatments might last for just a few minutes or longer. Some responses have been quite dramatic, while others have observed no differences. A negative static magnetic field appears "to destroy bacterial, fungal, and viral infections," calms the person for sleep, and normalizes enlarged areas of the body caused by fluid retention.

Veterinary research is more advanced in the use of magnets with animals than the allopathic community, but pain reduction is about the same in humans with arthritis as it appears to be in horses. There has been a noted improvement in healing of the tissues and nerves while having decreased healing times for tendons and bones. So for all the treatments used in horses, the pulsed magnetic flow has the same or better statistics for relieving pain, reducing swelling, controlling inflammation, and speeding healing as compared to the permanent, or static, magnets.

In animals, magnetic therapy initially appears to cause an overproduction of fibrous connective tissue and delays calcification on fresh fractures. After about two weeks from the time of injury, the magnets appear to support the healing process (i.e., enhance calcification). If there is a fresh wound or bruise, using magnets appears to result in excessive bleeding so waiting twenty-four to forty-eight hours before using them is prescribed. Caution should also be expressed with the use of magnets on acutely inflamed joints and open infected wounds, unless the low-frequency pulsed electromagnetic therapy is used.

The magnetic flow or pattern in the various wraps or pads is different from what is found in the standard magnet. In the standard magnet, the flow is from one end to the other. The patterned magnet materials contain grids that keep the magnetism from going to the edges and being "lost in space." Consumers are using these products to get relief for everything from joint and back pain to headaches and muscle spasms.

There is little research on the use of magnets and diabetes, but a number of people with neuropathy have reported to me that the shoe inserts have made life more bearable for them.

Magnetic therapy, too, has a long history. Its use comes from the cultures of Greece, China, India, and Egypt.

There are cautions: magnet therapy should not be used on pregnant women. Don't sleep on a magnetic bed for more than eight hours. Don't wear a magnet continuously. Wait an hour or so after a meal before applying a magnet. Positive magnetic pole treatment should not be used without the supervision of a physician.*

Call the Bio-Electro-Magnetics Institute at 702-827-9099 for more detailed information.

Thought Field Therapy (TFT)

"Practice is the best of all instructors." —*Publilius Syrus*

Thought field therapy offers training for people who want to eliminate fears and phobias and to handle concerns more rapidly. Dr. Roger Callahan, a psychologist, originated this approach. Thought field therapy works for the aspects of the thought field which contain the necessary information to trigger negative emotions. The stimulation of specific points along the meridians (not unlike those found in traditional Chinese medicine) promotes electromagnetic energy that impacts the thought field.

Such a simple activity as tapping below the eyes and tapping the outside edge of the hands can be used to speed up reading and comprehension. It was developed to treat not only phobias, but also depression, anxiety, traumatic stress, addictions, and other conditions. For instance, you're having trouble taking shots. A therapist could show you (or you could do it yourself) the tapping procedure to do before you take the shot. Not only would you find yourself less focused on the shot, but the whole procedure would also be perceived as being less threatening.

This is a noninvasive approach based on acupressure/acupuncture meridians. The learned self-treatments may stop the sequence of the electrical signals that are interpreted as problems. It has been shown to alter the autonomic nervous system. To get further information, you may call Dorothy Goertz, a nurse practitioner and clinical nurse specialist in psychiatric mental health, certified in TFT, at 316-367-2744, or for training in the Callahan Techniques, call 760-564-1008.

Pain Management Therapy

Pain management includes a variety of medicines and techniques, including thought field therapy. Many people overuse pain relievers (i.e., pills), so that when they are really needed, the relief is lessened, as the body has been conditioned to respond to chronic use. Certain over-the-

---

*These cautions are those listed in *Alternative Medicine: the Definitive Guide,* complied by The Burton Goldberg Group.

counter painkillers cause the production of excess acid in the stomach, leading to nausea, and vomiting, and result in increased susceptibility to the development of ulcers. Long-term use of pain relief has been associated with decreased blood clotting. Too high a dose of any over-the-counter product for pain may be toxic to the kidneys and liver.

The information included in this and the next section, at least, give alternatives to pill taking that do not injure the person in the process. These over-the-counter products are useful and have their place, but they should not be used indiscriminately.

The choices in pain management include, but are not limited to, aromatherapy, magnetic therapy, therapeutic touch, acupressure and acupuncture, hypnosis, guided imagery, hydrotherapy, chiropractic, biofeedback training, various massage techniques, nutrition and neural therapy (anesthetics injected into the nerve site). If a pill or injection is needed, especially for acute conditions, there is no doubt that it should be used. Especially in chronic situations, look for the therapy or herb that has the least side effects on a long-term and short-term basis.

If you have pain from neuropathy, consider the following:

1. Get a therapeutic massage.
2. Maintain blood sugars as normal as possible.
3. Keep active—walk whenever possible.
4. If surgery is suggested, get a second opinion.
5. If you are smoking, STOP.
6. Explore the use of alternative or complementary care, such as the use of capsicum (cayenne pepper) cream on tingling, burning feet.
7. Do things to get your mind off the discomfort.
8. Be referred to a pain center.

Be sure you and your health-care provider learn about the possible causes of the pain so that if anything can be remedied, such as a pinched nerve in the spine, it should be.

SELF-MANAGEMENT FOR DIABETES CONTROL

Self-management involves self-help. It also involves touch—not necessarily the kind you like, but it is there nevertheless. Touch is involved in testing your blood sugar. Contact is involved in checking your feet. Self-management involves making educated choices (developed with your health professional) in your daily regimen. Taking a medication, or administering an injection, or caring for your feet are all self-care practices.

Everyone hopes someday to be able to monitor blood glucose levels without having to pierce the skin. Did you know that a device has been developed and approved by the FDA to use with insulin infusion pumps? One is forthcoming that pierces the skin, but you don't have to use your fingers (or earlobes) but can use clear fluid from the cells on your finger or arm instead. There is also a lancing device (the Vaculance) that can use any part of your body that is less sensitive than your fingers. (Call about the Vaculance at 800-348-8100.) The only drawback is that you would need, unless you choose the finger as a site, a meter or strip that responds to "capillary action." This means that the blood is drawn up into the glucose test strip rather than you having to put a drop of blood on a stick (e.g., Glucometer Elite, Comfort Curve, At-Last).

A word of hope: there are more than eight companies testing noninvasive or continuous monitoring devices for blood glucose determinations.

Medication

Medications have not changed much; a new product, insulin that can be inhaled through the mouth, is a hope, once the testing process is complete. Insulin infusion pumps are becoming more refined. In fact, physicians have actually used these devices with infants, strapping the pump to the infant's back. These instruments are becoming more sophisticated and hopefully less expensive (right now, they add at least $2,000 per year to the total expenses of diabetes care).

More oral and injectable medications are on the way. Testing stages are needed before final approval is granted by the Food and Drug Administration, but other designer insulins are being worked on. By just changing the sequence of amino acids (or proteins) on the chain that forms the insulin, the outcome is an insulin that absorbs more rapidly or less rapidly.

As you feel able, and in coordination with your health professional, learn self-management. Your health professional cannot live with you twenty-four hours a day, but with self-management skills, you can make some of the changes within certain parameters and keep up with the changing needs of your body.

Food

Yes, you can change the insulin or medication at times, but consider altering the food. You would need more food for increased activity and would need less food for decreased activity.

When working toward normalizing blood sugars, as your blood glucose levels become more normal, recognize that you need less food to meet your metabolic needs (even just a few teaspoons to a few tablespoons less of each serving on your plate could help "shrink" your stomach to its new, healthier status). Note that if you eat much more than you need, the excess food will contribute not only to higher blood sugars but also to weight gain.

Checking Feet

Checking your feet is a chore for some individuals. If you have trouble seeing the bottom of your feet, try using an army or camping mirror. There are also adjustable inspection mirrors that can help with the routine of checking your feet for any signs of infection or pressure.

Hemoglobin A_{1c} Control

> "Sometimes, only a change of viewpoint is needed to convert a tiresome duty into an interesting opportunity."
> —*Alberta Flanders*

Work to get your hemoglobin A_{1c} below 7 percent or less than one percent above the upper limit of the laboratory's normal range, your blood pressure below 130/85 mm/hg, and your low-density lipoprotein level below 100 mg, especially if coronary heart disease is present. Cholesterol should be less than 200 mg, with the high-density lipoprotein higher than 35.

Be sure that the annual visit to the doctor includes a thorough neurological exam and a laboratory assessment of your kidneys, liver, microalbumin (a urine test if protein is not found in your urine by standard dipstick), lipids, complete blood count, thyroid tests (if symptomatic), and heart (electrocardiogram [ECG] if appropriate). Also recommended is yearly retinal eye exam (right after diagnosis for people with Type 2 diabetes and after five years of diagnosis for those with Type 1 diabetes) and a twenty-four-hour urine test for those individuals demonstrating protein in the urine to determine the rate of the urine going through the kidney (creatinine clearance).

Obtain continuing education about diabetes at least every two years if not more frequently. If you are planning to get pregnant, have your diabetes in control first. Keep up with your immunizations and, unless you're allergic to the shots, obtain the yearly flu shot. Continue to manage your weight and monitor your blood glucose levels. Look for patterns that either direct you to predict what changes you need, or change what is needed before the occurrence.

Look for ways to handle the stressors in your life. Use some form of stress management daily, including some form of increased activity. Exercise in some way no less than thirty minutes total per day, a minimum of three times a week. And see your doctor three to four times a year.

Just for Fun

"Don't do something because you have diabetes, do something safely and effectively in spite of having diabetes."
—*Guthrie and Guthrie*

Have you ever put cooled, green tea bags or slices of cucumber on your eyes, or mixed ground-up peaches with oatmeal and put this on your face as a mask for about ten minutes? Enhance this ten-minute wait by listening to some soothing music.

The combination of low cost, ease of availability, calming effect, safety, and health for the skin and eyes represents the ideal complementary therapy.

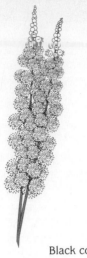

Black cohosh
(Cimiafuga racemosa)

9

TOUCH AND NONTOUCH REMEDIES

"We shall see but a little way if we are required to understand what we see." —*Henry David Thoreau*

Mike was experiencing terribly painful polyneuropathy. It involved the entire surface of his whole body. He said he almost wished he could just take his clothes off, as he was uncomfortable with them even touching his skin.

His physician was aiding him in normalizing his blood sugars. From the few blood sugar tests he had monitored, he reported that Mike's blood glucose levels had been abnormal for over four years.

Six months ago he had been diagnosed as having neuropathy in his feet. As his control improved, his feet hurt more. Then this "whole body" thing happened. He and I discussed how neuropathy affects the body. The positive piece of information was that this type of neuropathy could be reversed in nine months to a year, once blood glucose control was reestablished. The news he did not want to hear was that over these next months, as the blood sugars improved and some nerves regrew (new nerve growth is much more sensitive), he might feel even worse.

I challenged him with attaining and maintaining normal blood glucose levels as much of the time as possible in spite of any discomfort felt. To him, "pain was gain." Pain was reframed to represent the possibility that this complication was reversing.

We worked with biofeedback-enhanced relaxation training and self-hypnosis techniques. He learned techniques to be able to relax at will, along with putting himself into a trance-like state for specific periods of time.

During the therapy sessions I also used therapeutic touch and some other techniques of healing touch. His wife became proficient in giving therapeutic touch at home after a few short education sessions in the office.

The results? He learned to experience the relaxed, less painful periods as being much longer than they actually were. If he needed reinforcement about what he had learned, he could call if he was unable to get in for a clinic visit. He learned to feel at peace during times of greater discomfort.

The pain from the neuropathy gratefully lasted only about eight months. He states he still uses some of the skills he learned when he is stressed-out. He and his wife say they exchange therapeutic touch sessions for "any reason."

His self-care practices are now some of the best reported that I have heard. He said he didn't want to go through anything similar to that again. Out of the bad came the good. He felt better than he could remember feeling for a long, long time.

You have read about many new approaches to a variety of situations throughout this book. This chapter opens up an even larger field of choices that you might make to enhance the quality of your present lifestyle. The only guidelines in your choice or choices are how they "fit" you as a person in relation to your present health status, and to focus on the safety of their use.

THE USE OF TOUCH

If the body is out of balance, it does not function well. Traditional Chinese and Ayurveda medicine, as do a number of other modalities, attempt to help you attain and maintain a balance. Remember that conventional medicine focuses on illness as a result of a single problem and attempts to control this problem as a cure. In traditional Chinese medicine, there is a web of balancing influences on the body that include the physical, the emotional, genetics, and outside stressors. No two people are treated the same way, even if their presenting symptoms are the same. Not only the symptoms are examined but also any potential underlying causes related to one's patterns of eating, sleeping, and emotionally interacting with others.

Tibetan medicine has been brought to our Western eyes recently. This therapy distinguishes between the body and the mind, or soul, of the person, but does not treat these separately. Illness is thought to be a result of harmful behavior. The person must correct or avoid this harmful behavior to avoid future illnesses. Diagnosis is made by feeling the pulses (there are forty-eight different kinds).

To reestablish a balance, the therapist might suggest different ways of eating or different ways of considering the food that you eat. For instance, if you were to consider taste, note the following. There are fifty-seven different types of tastes when the following are used alone or in combination: sweet, sour, bitter, salty, astringent, and hot. Or you might consider the eight potencies (heat, coolness, sharpness, bluntness, coarseness, lightness, heaviness, and mildness). Herbs may be used alone or in combination (4 to 165 combinations) with massage, bleeding, cauterization, moxibustion, or other modalities. The physician, especially if Buddhist, may pray and meditate while administrating treatment. Rituals are used to play an important role, even if a specific therapy is not given (the placebo effect).

The first conference in the United States on Tibetan medicine was held during the fall of 1998. There is a film on Tibetan medicine completed in the 1990s. For information on showings of the film in the United States, call 212-925-5656.

Acupuncture

Acupuncture treatment must be given by a certified or licensed practitioner. This is not a therapy that you would do yourself. It is the placing of very fine needles in the meridian points (energy points) related to the areas of need.

When you go to the office of an acupuncturalist or a health professional trained in these practices, you will be intensely questioned about your total life practices. Your pulses might be palpated and your tongue examined. A plan is developed and the treatment begins.

The needles, hair thin, will be inserted at various depths at sites related to the twelve main meridians (there are more than a thousand acupoints).

Heat (moxibustion) or electricity might be applied to the end of the needle. Cupping (or suction) might be applied once the needle is removed in order to increase the circulation.

Discomfort, in most instances, will be little or none. The needles are usually kept in place for twenty to thirty minutes.

The majority of acupuncturists work in cooperation with Western medicine, so that any modification in medication dosages or other treatments will be weighed in the plan. Risk is little, so long as the skin is clean and the needles are not contaminated. Make sure that disposable needles are used.

The use of acupuncture, a more-than-two-thousand-year-old practice, might be continued even if no noticeable change occurred. The diagnosis might change, but the treatment might remain the same because of the original holistic assessment.

The professional use of acupuncture has resulted in forty colleges offering courses in acupuncture and twenty-nine states offering licensure. Acupuncture appears to be moderately effective in the treatment of arthritis, acute back pain, chronic low-back pain, whiplash injury, chronic neck pain, tension headaches, dysmenorrhea (painful menstrual periods), irritable bowel syndrome, and sinus headaches. Research supports its use for pain and anxiety, and it is now being tested for its affect on depression. People who have diabetes might find it helpful when experiencing painful symptoms not controlled by standard practices or as an alternative to taking pain medicine. The success rate is about 70 percent. Although it may not work immediately, once the effect is experienced, it may last for weeks or more after the treatments have been concluded. If no change is experienced in six sessions, you might want to try something else.

How acupuncture works is still being researched. Whether it interrupts the gate pathways for pain or stirs up the release of chemicals called endorphins (similar to morphine biochemically), pain is lessened or even eliminated.

In the 1960s, Kim Bong Han, a professor, and others found, using microdissection techniques, evidence that there is an independent series of fine duct-like tubes corresponding to the meridians. Fluids in these tubes were found to flow in the same and also in the opposite direction as the blood and lymph.

A French researcher, Pierre de Vernejoul, injected radioactive isotopes and then tracked their movement with a gamma-imaging camera. He found that the isotopes did not travel in the same manner when placed in the blood versus being placed in the meridians.

In the 1970s, the National Institutes of Health funded Dr. Robert Becker and Maria Reichmanis, who were able to prove that electrical currents did indeed flow along the meridians and that the acupuncture points did exist.

Another point of information: it is known that acupuncture stimulates the release of endorphins, more popularly associated with exercise, as discoverd by Dr. David Eisenberg at Harvard Medical School. Since endorphins biochemically closely resemble morphine, the pain relief is a little more understandable.

Auriculotherapy, or ear acupuncture, may also be used for most of the same conditions as for the rest of the body. Such things as ear massage and electrical stimulation have also been successful in treating various maladies.

The World Health Organization said that there are 104 different conditions that acupuncture can treat, including pain, addictions, mental disorders, and AIDS. The United States House of Representatives and Senate found that acupuncture for substance abuse is cost-effective and should be used widely.

Choose an acupuncture specialist by recommendation and/or credentials. The American Association of Acupuncture and Oriental Medicine may be reached by calling 919-787-5181.

Acupressure

Acupressure also focuses on healing, and is used to remove trapped energy and allow the flow of the life force, or *qi* (pronounced *chi*). When *qi* flows smoothly, that means good health is present. Acupressure has been found most useful in treating nausea and vomiting, headaches and backaches. There are acupressure points on either side of the middle of the upper spine that are useful in relieving hiccups.

There are self-acupressure techniques. They are called Acu-Yoga and Do-In. Acu-Yoga uses whole body breathing along with pressure on specific points, the yoga postures, the yoga stretches, and meditation. On the other hand, Do-In, while using stretching and breathing, focuses more on body awareness and the stimulation of the body through the pressure points and meridians.

Acupressure should be avoided near the abdominal area of pregnant women. It is also not recommended to do any acupressure near varicose veins or bones or wounds.

The history of writings about acupressure and, later, acupuncture go back 4,500 years. The first books of *Nie Ching* took about 1,500 years to complete. Acupressure massage involves the use of rubbing, kneading, percussion, and vibration for stimulation of the energy meridians and acupressure points. This process is called Tui Na in China and Amma in Japan.

Some acupressure points that you might find useful are the ones for headache (in the corner space between the thumb and second finger, and on the felt "notch" at the top of the inner aspect of the eyeball socket, and one and a half or so inches from the center of the head with pressure on the occipital bones); behind the ankle bone on the outer aspect of the foot or three fingers up from the ankle bone (on the outside of the leg) for ankle and foot discomfort; four inches below the navel for constipation; pressure halfway between the end of the nose and the upper edge of the lip for control of fainting; treat hiccups by putting pressure on the inner aspect of the second joint of the third finger, or midway down the back, about one to two inches on either side of the spine (lower end of the seventh thoracic vertebra); treat motion sickness by putting pressure two inches up from the middle of the end of the palm; and treat sinus pain or congestion by putting pressure on the bone on both sides or either side adjacent to the edge of the openings of the nose.

You are pressing on the right spots if there is a tingling (electrical) sensation. The pressure must be firm and in a small circular massage motion but not enough to result in bruising of the skin. The length of time might be from one to five minutes.

If you find some of these points helpful, pick up an acupressure book and learn more. Be sure to recognize that in most instances, pain is an indication of a problem, and if persistent, you should have it assessed by a health professional. The Acupressure Institute may be contacted for information and training at 510-845-1059; the American Association of

Acupuncture and Oriental Medicine may be reached by calling 919-787-5181.

Ayurveda—Foods/Water

Ayurvedic medicine is considered the oldest medical system known. *Ayurveda* is Sanskrit for "the science of life." The *constitution* is the word used to refer to the overall health profile of the person. Dr. Deepak Chopra is responsible for popularizing the practice of Ayurveda in this country.

This approach was transplanted into India with the arrival of the Aryan invaders. It practices a rebalancing of hot and cold, yin and yang, etc., and illness is seen as the absence of harmony of the physical, emotional, and spiritual aspects of the person. The unbalancing of the person is believed to be based on seven major factors: genetics, congenital problems, internal and external trauma, season of the year, magnetic and electrical influences, and natural tendencies or habits. These practitioners also question the patient intensely and then look at the tongue and evaluate the pulses.

Traditional Chinese medicine considers the ear as a model for the inverted body and associated organs, whereas Ayurveda considers the tongue: heart, lungs (right and left) at the tip to middle; spleen, stomach, liver, and pancreas to the middle; and intestines and left and right kidney to the back, with the left and right being associated with the left and right orientation of the observer.

Other techniques that might be used in the evaluation also include inspection of the nails and lips and the other orifices of the body. Treatment consists not only of breathing exercise, but also of developing a way of eating and taking care of the body through massage and elimination and purification, and meditating to balance the spiritual aspect of the person.

Being identified as one of the three metabolic types, or *doshas,* influences the plan for that person. *Kapha* is the heavy person; *pitta* is the medium-size person, and *vata* is the slender or thinner person.

Ayurvedic medicine, like traditional Chinese medicine, uses herbs in the balancing process and considers the elements of earth, water, fire, metal, and wood. Each of the *doshas* is "responsible" for the body's various functions associated with these elements.

Purging, according to ancient practice, is at times still done, i.e., *pancha karma*. This could involve applying leeches, inducing vomiting, nasal washing, or bowel purging. Specific herbs, medicated oils, and ghee (a butter) are used as a nasal wash to increase mental clarity.

After the *pancha karma* is completed, the person is directed to palliation or "shaman." This is used to rebalance the body. It might include a fast, exercise (yoga), meditation, breathing exercises, hot herbs, or the person might be directed to get fresh air by lying outside. Some heavy metals are used in their traditional medicine, but this use is not condoned in the United States. Yoga, or "union" (the science of the spirit), is frequently used with Ayurveda (the science of the body).

This regimen is followed by *rasayana,* or rejuvenation. This is done by ingesting special herbs, using mineral preparations, and the use of exercises (more yoga and other breathing exercises).

Satvajaya is a process used for spiritual healing. This works on the emotional as well as the spiritual side of care. It includes a mantra or sound therapy to change the vibratory patterns of the mind, concentration to change the way one thinks, and meditation to alter states of consciousness. Gems, metals, and crystals maybe be used for their subtle vibratory healing power.

An uncontrolled study (no comparison group) of 149 people who had diabetes concluded that the use of yoga therapy decreased blood glucose levels and, therefore, showed less need of diabetes medications. At the time of the study, the subjects were placed on a vegetarian diet, and that alone could have influenced the outcome.

Ayurveda is a self-care practice program; the individual is given a lot of instruction so that he/she will follow through on the practices introduced during the therapeutic session. A good source of information may be obtained from the Sharp Institute for Human Potential and Mind-Body Medicine (800-82-SHARP).

Shiatsu

Shiatsu comes from the Japanese word *shi* ("finger") and *atsu* ("pressure") or "finger pressure." It is a technique that originated in Japan about seventy years ago but is based on Chinese medical theories that were introduced into Japan a thousand or so years ago.

Shiatsu is often considered as a type of massage, when in actuality, it is a form of acupressure. Shiatsu and acupressure are often mentioned together. Acupressure is the older of the techniques when compared to acupuncture. It may involve more massage movements than shiatsu, while shiatsu may involve more body manipulations and movements with its use of finger pressure.

There are many different schools of shiatsu in Japan. There is the classic or brusque style, the more popular softer approach, and the barefoot style. Its use is based on the philosophy that the body has its own healing powers. Shiatsu assists in discovering the cause of illness or discomfort. The result is that a person might actually initially feel worse from the treatment because of the unbalancing as a result of the initial assessment and sensitivity to the pressure on certain points in the body. The focus is again to rebalance the body by pressing on about 90 of the 361 *tsubos,* or small indentations, under the skin.

Diagnosis is then noted through observation (*Do-shin*), through sound (*Bun-shin*), through questioning (*Mon-shin*), and through touch (*Setsu-shin*). This last part is actually diagnosis (*hara*) through touch. All energy comes and goes through the *hara* (where the yin and yang meet). Disease is thought to come from the *hara* or the body's center of gravity.

The two main techniques are gentle stretching while rotating with pressure a body part at the joint. This pressure may be applied by fingertips, palms, elbows, and toes. The pressure and movement is downward and vertical. A specific sequence of pressure to identified points is held for three to ten seconds. The breathing of the practitioner should synchronize with that of the client. The yellow pages of the phone book, under massage, often list the types of massage performed by a shiatsu therapist.

Therapeutic Touch

This again is a distinctive therapy involving energy flow. Therapeutic touch is the outcome of the skills of Dora Kuntz and the research of Professor Delores Krieger. Dr. Krieger says she was influenced by the skills of Dora Kuntz and the practices of yoga, Ayurvedic, Tibetan, and Chinese health systems. The transfer of energy is based on Asian and Indian therapies.

There may or may not be physical touch between the therapist and the client. The client is asked to lie down or sit in a chair that is most comfortable. The clothes remain in place. A blanket might be placed over the client's body from the neck down if the room is chilly or if the client desires. The procedure is as follows:

The simple steps are: centering (or focusing on the client and the client's needs); assessing (or determining sites of the body that need therapeutic intervention); unruffling (or clearing the energy field); intervention (or balancing the energy field); and reassessment (or determining if further intervention is needed). This is usually done with the hand about four inches or so above the body, palms down.

Blocks in energy flow are usually sensed by a feeling of coldness. Infection or excess energy is noted by a feeling of warmth. Congestion is felt as variations in sensations experienced by the hands. The practitioner works with the client until these areas all feel similar, i.e., no area is hotter, colder, or more congested than another. The average treatment lasts about twenty minutes more or less.

Dr. Krieger states that therapeutic touch or TT is "a contemporary interpretation of several ancient healing practices in which the practitioners consciously direct or sensitively modulate (intervention) human energies." It is used in many hospitals and clinics as a way to calm, reduce pain, and put the body into a state of quiet.

Multiple research studies have shown that TT can alter enzyme activity, increase the hemoglobin in red blood cells, and speed the healing of wounds, along with decreasing pain and anxiety. It is considered closely related to the concept of laying on of hands, practiced by ministers of several faiths. Rather than being religiously based, the power of TT is related to the idea of energy fields within and around the body.

A recent study reported in the *New England Journal of Medicine,* performed by an eleven-year-old girl, had the outcome that TT did not work. The girl's parents were opposed to any type of energy therapy, and the eleven-year-old most likely was influenced by her parents' biases. The intent was not there, and whatever energy blocking occurred as she randomly held her hand over the arm of a "blinded" TT therapist who was to tell her if she was "present" or not, interfered with the process significantly. Specialists in the subtle energy field, along with the Nurse Healers Professional Association International, responded by identifying the problems associated with the study and the bias of the "researcher."

Other research on TT (over forty-seven studies) does show that it has an effect on both humans and animals. It was seen to have a calming effect on children and to decrease anxiety in hospitalized patients. Healing of wounds in mice was found to be faster (a study done by the Canadian healer Oskar Estabany). The need for pain medications appears to be less when TT is used.

For more information and location of courses (Dr. Krieger feels that all people can be taught this technique), call 703-437-4377.

Healing Touch

Healing touch is a therapeutic approach used to influence the energy system of the body. Its goal is to affect the physical, emotional, mental, and spiritual well-being of the client. It is an approach that rebalances and restores harmony through the rebalancing and restoration of the harmony in the energy system.

The program was developed by Janet Mentgen in the late 1970s. The multilevel energy-based program is also open to any who wish to learn.

It includes such techniques as therapeutic touch, penduluming, hand scanning, magnetic unruffling, chakra connection, headache technique, a technique called ultrasound, one called the chakra spread, and the Scudder technique. Other techniques are learned as the participant progresses through three levels for certification and the fourth level if he/she wishes to be involved in instruction.

Through the practitioner using various techniques, the client is aided in the intent to restore wholeness. It is noninvasive and complements other approaches to the improvement of health. Consideration is given to the layers of the energy field or aura. These layers are etheric (0.25 to 2 inches from the body); the emotional field (from one to three inches beyond the surface of the body); the mental field (extending three to eight inches), and the spiritual field (made up of four or more layers which extend to about twenty-four inches or more from the body).

Energy centers or chakras (a Sanskrit word meaning "wheel" or "disklike") connect with lines or energy tracts called meridians within the energy field or aura. As noted with other energy modalities, these energy effects relate to the nervous and endocrine systems.

Chakras can be assessed through the use of the pendulum: little or no motion noted in the pendulum indicates a blocked chakra; full movement of the pendulum in a clockwise direction indicates an open chakra. A specific technique is taught to both open and close these chakras or the chakra connections. Levels of energy above the body are experienced through the sensitive use of the hands.

A woman was my partner in the session on sensing the energy levels of a person's aura. All was going well (i.e., I could sense a different resistance when reaching another layer) until I came to the second or sacral chakra. I thought I had done something wrong, so I tried again. As soon as my hands were over the lower part of the abdomen, "there was nothing there" (there was no feeling of resistance or energy flow).

In the debriefing session afterward, I found that this person had experienced some trauma earlier in life and was attempting to come to terms with this problem even at this time. The blockage was there at this chakra level. She felt it. I felt it.

Healing touch represents a world that is interdependent, one person and that environment on the other person and environment. All things are affected by energy. Action and thought influence the ability of a person to be healed through integrated energy. For more information see the *Healing Touch Level I/II Notebooks* by Janet Mentgen and Mary Jo Trapp Bulbrook of Healing Touch International (303-989-0581).

Reiki

Reiki is a technique concerned with moving energy through the body to keep the body's balance. Reiki therapy has a most fascinating history. Some say it was developed by a Japanese businessman, but a more authentic story follows:

A Japanese doctor of theology, monk, and educator, Dr. Mikao Usui, was questioned in 1850 by his students, "If Jesus said, follow me, he was to be the example—and he healed people. Then why can't we heal people, too?" The professor reflected much on this point and traveled all over the world to find a "healing process." He tried many modalities but was not satisfied with his experiences. On returning to Japan, he went on retreat—finding himself quite disappointed in not getting an answer to the question. Then, as he told it, he was literally hit with an energy power that knocked him off his feet. The answer he sought was there. The energy from heaven would travel through the practitioner and to the recipient.

He then set about refining the process, in the 1800s, as he worked with many individuals and assisted them in their return to health. Various techniques and positions of the hand placement on the body are taught in order to connect the energy flow and increase your energy supply. Symbols are used as healing and communication devices as the practitioner increases in skills and in levels of training.

Level one involves the history, concepts, and hands-on practices. On the second level, distance therapy is learned. Level three is needed to become a master practitioner (some programs have other levels).

The position of Reiki master is achieved through working with a mentor for several years. This includes learning how to teach Reiki along with self-growth through self-reflection.

Masters are also taught how to initiate others into the discipline. These series for the learner have the purpose of balancing and fine-tuning the students' own energy fields.

Reiki requires the learning of formalized hand positions (ten hand positions for the front and eight hand positions on the back—held in each position for four to five minutes). It does not require an assessment of the body before proceeding. It is noninvasive.

As with healing touch and therapeutic touch, Reiki is considered an energy-based modality. Research appears to support that Reiki works by affecting the neuroendocrine system, but double-blind studies as to its actual effect need to be completed.

There are some controversies as to the exact and correct method of approach to the energy therapy and healing process. Though the skills learned might depend on the Reiki master and vary somewhat, they all appear to be focused toward the same goal. There are reports of different effects on different people. Read the phenomenological (a what happened) study by Ahlam Mansour and others, in the June 1998 issue (pages 211 to 217), of *Alternative and Complementary Therapies.*

Jin Shin Jyutsu

Jin Shin Jyutsu has recently become more popular. It is another Oriental body work that shares some of the same principles—such as rebalancing the body's energy—of acupuncture and Oriental medicine.

This modality was developed in Japan by Jiro Murae. The client is prone on a padded table or bed. The therapist presses, with fingertips, on a combination of points until a balance in the pulses is felt. Variations of this style include Jin Shin Tara, Jin Shin Do, and Jin Shin acupressure. All of these modalities are based on the belief that a person has the capacity to heal though touch.

These techniques can be used for stress reduction or as an approach to harmonize the body for the potential of healing. Stress reduction should promote the stabilization of blood glucose levels.

BODY WORK

Any type of body work appears to have some effect on the body. From the massage of a tiny infant to the realignment of an elderly person's posture, a sense of calm and serenity appear to be common outcomes. Massage enhances the flow of blood and relaxes the muscles that are tense.

A choice of a specific body work activity, such as massage, might just relieve pain, or it might also energize you. If it is actually improving blood flow to various parts of the body or rebalancing body functions, it might be just what you need. The following descriptions of types of body work will help you choose among them—whether you want help with a specific need or just want to relax.

Craniosacral Massage

John Upledger, an osteopathic physician, has written numerous books and articles on this subject, even though its original developer, in the 1900s, was Dr. William G. Sutherland, an osteopath. Dr. Sutherland focused this therapy on the bones of the head, spine, and pelvis (that is, cranio = head; sacral = base of the spine).

The purpose of craniosacral massage is to increase the pressure of the flow of the cerebrospinal fluid. This therapy is thought to be useful for people of all ages, but some pediatricians have had concerns about its use in children due to their softer bones, especially in early infancy. The basic premise is that what you do on the head will influence the cerebrospinal fluid pressure. The scientific question is whether the skull's separate bones can actually be moved, as most texts teach that these are nonmovable in the adult human scull.

This type of therapy is thought to be useful in treating chronic pain, epilepsy, tinnitus, and edema, among others. It is also reported to be useful in treating headaches. Since it is nonintrusive, it may be helpful, but if it is used in instances when other approaches should be considered (for example, a severe headache caused by a brain tumor), it could be harmful (for instance, used in place of early therapy that might shrink or remove the tumor). Successes have been based on reports by people participating in such massage. Actual comparative studies are needed. For more information, contact the various schools of associated thought: Cranial Academy (Dr. William Sutherland's work) at 317-879-0713; Dr. Major DeJarnette's work at SORSI 913-649-3475; or the Upledger Institute at 407-622-4706.

Feldenkrais Method—Person in Motion

This is an approach that is associated with "awareness through movement," and "functional integration," as developed by Moshe Feldenkrais, a physicist. His focus was on self-awareness and movement rather than on manipulative massage. He founded this approach, as did others, as a result of his own injuries and his wish not to use traditional methods.

This approach, individualized for each patient, either guides a person through a sequence of movements, or uses hands-on techniques. These are thought to support not only movement of body parts but also improvement of self-image. An example might be the movement of only the arms by a guide or by the patient in a specific direction for a comfortable number of times. This would be followed by imagining the same movement with even increased awareness of smoothness of movement and increased distance of movement. The next step would be to actually repeat the movement and note the improved flow of movement and increased range of movement. This is useful for sports participation improvement and improvement after healing from trauma (800-775-2118; www.feldenkrais.com).

Reflexology

Some people swear by their reflexologist. Reflexogy is a technique to assess and alter various responses in the body as identified by pressure on various points of the feet. Having your feet massaged is beneficial, but further information through the therapist's contact with your feet gives added value to the session. Just as traditional Chinese medicine partially relies on points of the ear to represent various parts of the anatomy, so does reflexology contend that various points on the hands and feet represent various organs and parts of the body. While the work on these points is supposed to relieve tension, the improved blood flow and energy unblocking aids in improved functioning of that part of the body.

"Unblocking" energy flow is a goal. Tenderness at a site on the foot indicates a potential problem to that associated part of the body. Pressure on that spot leads to unblocked energy.

Foot massage is often given at an introduction and at the completion of a session. During the session itself, pressure is, as noted before, focused on what are called "reflex points." This therapy can be performed by you. But it does take training to do it correctly, by applying pressure to the reflex points of need especially for the thirty minutes or more of the "treatment."

Dr. William Fitzgerald initially developed a therapy through his findings as an otolaryngologist (ear and throat specialist). By applying pressure to certain parts of the mouth and hands he was able to obtain numbness and/or other responses in the face. A physiotherapist and nurse named Eunice Ingham expanded Fitzgerald's work and was responsible for mapping these reflex areas in the body through her work on the feet and hands.

The scientific research studies that have been carried out note both questionable and positive outcomes. No matter what the outcomes, so long as reflexology is not relied on for any diagnostic purposes for treatment for specific ailments, it does appear to be a safe way to decrease tension and give some relief of pain.

For more information, call the International Institute of Reflexology at 813-343-4811.

Rolfing—Person Standing Straight

Ida Rolf, a biochemist, was influenced by chiropractic treatment and hatha yoga. She founded the "home" of Structural Integration, also known as Rolfing. Rolfing is re-balancing or realigning the body. It is achieved by releasing adhesions though massage and movement of specific identified areas. Therapists are taught to use any part of their hands, their knees, and/or their elbows in this process of releasing fascial (muscle) adhesions during weekly sessions (often ten sessions or more).

Research found that Rolfing improved movements of the body, especially the tilt of the pelvis. It actually was therapeutic in improving poor posture. But controlled (scientific) studies are still needed.

This technique is based on two premises: (1) fascia can harden over time; and (2) a misaligned body requires more energy to move. Their focus is not on curing, but on improving the quality of life. The massage relieves tension and thereby decreases stress levels. Call the Rolf Institute (303-499-5903) for more information on this modality.

Aston patterning and Hellerwork are variations on Dr. Rolf's work. Aston patterning involves education about movement in relation to the person's environment, as does Rolfing, along with a system of massage. Heller adds other exercises to the basic Rolfing technique.

Rosen Method

The Rosen method is rapidly becoming more popular. It combines massage with a quiet form of nondirective counseling that can be very therapeutic. It was developed by a physical therapist (Martha Rosen) when she observed a strong association between emotional tension and muscular tension.

In her work as an apprentice to Dr. Lucy Heyer, a psychotherapist, she learned about massage and breathing. She noted that patients who discussed their problems appeared to heal more quickly. It appeared that agitated emotions often resulted in tense muscles. Rosen released the emotions through the gentle art of massage.

As the muscles become more relaxed, the Rosen therapist will carry on a discussion with the client. This discussion will attempt to bring to the surface the emotions the person is experiencing. Often the revelation of such emotions appears to be therapeutic in and of itself. In other instances, just talking about the emotions has been found useful. If deeper issues are at stake, referral to another type of therapist would be recommended. In fact, this type of therapy is a good adjunct to psychotherapy.

The therapy starts with the client lightly clothed. The massage begins, without the use of oils, on the middle back (on top of the diaphragm). As the massage moves to various areas of the body, in time with the breathing (and observation of the type of breathing) of the client, the therapist gets the client to talk about potentially associated emotional blocks. These areas of discussion are guided by the therapist finding tension in various muscle groups and by the therapist noting changes in breathing patterns at various times during the conversation.

As you study more about this type of therapy, using such a therapy might assist you in unleashing and resolving the feelings you have about the diagnosis of diabetes mellitus. The Rosen Institute may be reached by calling 510-845-6606 or the Rosen Method Professional Association (510-644-4166) to find a therapist in your area and for more information about its use.

Swedish Massage

Therapeutic massage is considered body work. Previous types of specific bodywork have already been discussed, but generalized massage for general health and comfort will be included here. This full body massage was once taught to nursing students as part of their basic education program.

The history of therapeutic massage dates back about five thousand years. Per Henrik Ling, a physician in Sweden, developed this form of massage. Again, through the art of relaxing muscles, it also reduces stress. As stress responses are decreased, associated diseases, such as high blood pressure, depression, and diabetes, appear to be improved. Even Hippocrates, the ancient Greek physician, promoted the use of massage.

The physiology of massage (from the Arabic word "to stroke") is based on releasing lactic acid from tense muscles. This lactic acid results in soreness if not properly removed from the muscle cells. Massage is recognized as improving muscle flow, thereby theoretically aiding in the removal of lactic acid from the cells.

Swedish massage is based on five specific techniques. The long gliding strokes of "effleurage" usually are found at the beginning and end of the massage treatment. If you feel as if your muscles are being kneaded, not unlike bread dough, then you are receiving "petrissage." Deep circular movements are termed "friction." A fine shaking movement is called, "vibration." If you feel the rapid, alternate, but comfortable "beating" of the hands on a muscle, you are receiving "tapotement." This might be accomplished by using the outside edge of the hand, a tapping with the fingertips, the use of tight or loose fists, or a cupping of the hands.

These techniques may be used in sequence on various parts of the body or where the therapist feels they are needed. An oil, creme, or powder might be used. The therapist will usually ask you about your preference about using any type of scents before actually applying one to your skin.

Massage without such oils or powders is possible (i.e., deep massage), but the flow on the body parts may not be as smooth. Moist heat packs may be used to relax a muscle or muscles before the massage begins.

Therapeutic massage is usually accomplished on the properly draped, unclothed body. Massage on sensitive parts of the body are routinely omitted. Although there are some types of massage that are deeper (deep fascia massage), or lighter, the Swedish massage is usually vigorous and firm.

Sports massage is often thought of as similar to Swedish massage, but it involves only two techniques: kneading and range of motion. It is not uncommon that a therapist will be educated in both, and therefore, combine both types of massage.

FINAL COMMENTS

"Nothing is so strong as gentleness; and nothing is so gentle
as real strength." —*Ralph W. Stockman*

The research on massage is increasingly present in the literature. This includes research about children as well as adults. The approach to research has been based on physiological changes and quality of life or psychosocial changes.

Cautions include not massaging an infected site, an inflamed site or site of suspected inflammation of a blood vessel, or at a site of a recent injury. Determine if the massage therapist is certified. Prices for one half hour or full hour will vary in different parts of the country ($35 to $70 an hour are not uncommon). For locating a certified massage therapist in your community, contact the National Certification Board for Therapeutic Massage (800-296-0664).

Whatever form of body work you choose, it should be done in a quiet, clean environment with the therapist qualified to administer that particular type of program. Professionalism and individualism are the key concepts. As you find a therapist who treats you and your special needs in a respectful way, your comfort and therapeutic advantages from the use of that modality will be enhanced.

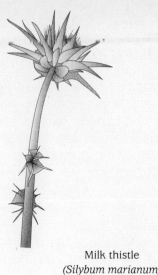

Milk thistle
(Silybum marianum)

10

NOW IT'S YOUR TURN

"Vision without action is a daydream. Action without vision
is a nightmare." —*Japanese proverb*

The National Institutes of Health's National Center for Complementary and Alternative Medicine defines complementary and alternative medicine as "those treatments and health care practices not taught widely in medical [or nursing] school, not generally used in hospitals, and not usually reimbursed by medical insurance companies." *Holistic* is defined by the American Holistic Nurses Association as any practice that focuses on healing the whole person as a goal—bodymindspirit (remember: these are all connected and interactive). Curing is the termination of a disease through surgical, chemical, or mechanical means.

Healing is a gradual awakening of a sense of self that results in readiness to grow and change.

These definitions are repeated to remind you of the importance of you as an individual who just happens to have diabetes. Because you have diabetes, extra care must be given when attempting to achieve a balance between your body, your mind, and your spirit. This chapter then is really the most important chapter in the book.

Learning about alternative and complementary therapies is one thing. Using these therapies wisely is another. (Good news! Capital University in Washington, D.C., graduated the first class in 1998 of physicians who completed a program in alternative and complementary education. Plans are to eventually have this course available to physicians in the Midwest and West Coast. The spring of 1999 saw the first graduates of the Integrative Medicine program under Dr. Andrew Weil, at the University of Arizona at Tucson.)

There is great potential in alternative and complementary care, but there is also danger if a choice is wrong for you. You may be frustrated when told there is no scientific evidence that proves a modality is beneficial. If a therapy (remember: for the sake of discussion this includes the use of vitamins, minerals, and herbs) has no or few reported side effects, be sure to find out if they mean on a short-term basis or for prolonged treatment. Accept that the therapy you choose might work for you and not for "your neighbor." It might work better when used with your prescribed regimen than when used alone. What you believe about a therapy might lead to a positive outcome for you.

For instance, you work with a remedy and find that your blood glucose levels are lower. If you are not taught self-management, be sure to contact your health professional for advice in lowering your traditional diabetes medicine. If you are taught self-management, then recognize that the time to decrease you medication is prior to the time of lowered blood sugar. Discuss such changes with your health professional at your next visit or by phone.

WHAT DO YOU NEED?

"You see things; and you say, 'Why?' But I dream
of things that never were; and I say, 'Why not?'"
—*George Bernard Shaw*

In a study released in the fall of 1998, Dr. Eisenberg and others reported that people paid an estimated $27 billion for alternative therapies.

Americans made about 629 million trips to alternative providers, compared with 386 million visits to primary care doctors.

The majority of the public does not recognize that basic dietary needs may usually be obtained by daily food intake only if you are eating whole foods grown in an adequate and naturally mineralized environment and your choice of foods is well balanced. If your lifestyle prevents you from eating correctly or you are following a weight-loss program of less than 1,200 calories, there is no doubt that supplements would be useful. Certainly, choices of supplements might include vitamins, minerals, herbs, and fiber. If you don't need the supplement and you have good working kidneys you will probably just excrete the excess in your urine. Megadoses may not be the best thing unless you are working with a knowledgeable person.

Not eating correctly means you are not taking the time needed for your own balanced health-care program or you are unable to do so because of a specific health problem. A hectic lifestyle is not a healthy lifestyle. Priorities exist no matter how stressful life might be. Perhaps you should be one of those people who recognizes that having to take supplements is a cue that you need to readjust your priorities, slow down, and take time to "smell the roses"—or find something that works. Since the most common use of alternative treatment is mostly to alleviate chronic conditions such as headaches, back or other pain, insomnia, anxiety, or depression, health professionals should get the message when what they are recommending is not working.

One study funded by Mutual of Omaha found that involvement in an exercise routine, meditation, support group, and a strict diet cost $5,500. This is quite a saving when compared to $40,000 for a heart bypass. From the standpoint of cost effectiveness alone, the company estimated it could save $6.50 for every dollar spent. This does not mean that the bypass should be discarded when medically needed, but it does mean prevention is more cost saving than treatment. Now other companies are asking "Why?" and are beginning their own studies.

Do your own self-assessment. Determine for yourself (or ask for help) what your lifestyle is doing to you and what is needed to assist you in being healthier.

ASK YOUR PHARMACIST

Of a large group of surveyed pharmacists, 100 percent said that consumers have asked them about herbal remedies. You need resources to study and to share with your health professional.

Self-Assessment

Name	Height	Weight	BMI	Age
Activity level:	High	Mod.	Low	
Stress level:	High	Mod.	Low	
24-hr. food history:	Breakfast:			
	Snack:			
	Lunch:			
	Snack:			
	Supper:			
	Snack:			
	Other:			
Sleep:	Time to bed	Time up at night	Time of Awakening	Time of Nap(s)
Quality of sleep:	Good	Mod	Poor	

Exercise/activity program (include frequency, intensity, time, and type):

All medications, including vitamins, minerals, and herbals:

Body works: (example: massage once a week)

Strengths of your program: _____

Weaknesses of your program: _____

Planned changes in program: _____

You may have already looked at the resources at the end of this book. These books are not gospel. They are there to add to your thinking, to your questioning, and to your decision-making process. Remember that too much or too little of anything can be a problem. Going "overboard" in trying a new approach, unless supported by adequate professional guidance could get you in trouble: from toxicity resulting from your body's inability to excrete a product because your kidneys or liver are not functioning properly, or resulting from your body responding with blood sugars that are too high or too low.

In the first place, recognize that if you have compromised (below the desired level of functioning) liver function, kidney function, or both, you could get into severe problems.

Intestinal absorption is another problem, especially if you have diabetic diarrhea or gastroparesis (bloating, etc). Too rapid an uptake could mean too fast a response to an herb, vitamin, or mineral. Too slow an uptake just usually means you've poured money down the drain. The same with water-soluble vitamins and herbs. What your body doesn't use it loses, or, as my husband says, "You'll end up feeding the fish."

Illness can occur through excess use of fat-soluble vitamins, or if your body has a total fat intake of less than 20 percent, which results if these vitamins are not being absorbed. If you are unable to release this excess of fat-soluble vitamins from your body as a waste product, you could become sick. The worst case scenario is that you will be hospitalized.

Vitamins, minerals, and herbs are considered dietary supplements. Remember that they are not regulated by the Food and Drug Administration or other organization as they are in Europe. If you experience problems with breathing, a skin rash, problems with diarrhea or a headache within two hours of taking an herb, stop taking it. You may be allergic to the herb (or vitamin or mineral) you have taken.

Look for the word *standardized* as nutritional information on the label. It means you're getting a specific amount of herb, vitamin, or mineral in each tablet, capsule, or tincture. If that word is not on the label, you have no idea as to its source, the consistency of amount in each portion, or the quality of the herb. This also means to steer clear of "secret formulas." You should know what is being recommended and why.

Don't be caught up by advertisements about miraculous cures. If it is too good to be true, it probably is. Basically, question everything. Don't take things at face value.

Mary is a twenty-four-year-old with Type 1 diabetes. She is trying to maintain her weight, eat correctly, and spend time daily or every other day working on exercises and flexibility. During her late teenage years she had many months of hemoglobin A_{1c} 9 percent or above. She has recently been diagnosed as having vascular problems and elevated cholesterol levels.

After much discussion and study with her physician, they have agreed to a trial use of daily pressed garlic capsules containing allicin (for cholesterol), and hawthorne (for its vascular lowering effect), along with intense control of blood glucose levels.

Six months later she was found to have hemoglobin A_{1c} of 7.2 percent, normal cholesterol, HDL, and LDL levels. Her most pleasing piece of news was the report from her physician that her blood vessels had somewhat improved from the previous diagnosed condition.

This is a person with Type 2 diabetes who also had a good response to his choices:

John completed his self-assessment. He has had Type 2 diabetes for eight years. He had a ten-year history of alcohol addiction and was celebrating his fourth dry year. His health-care provider felt that in his overweight stage he needed the addition of another oral agent to control his blood sugar. The medication the health professional wished to use was a metformin, but John's last multiple chemical profile revealed some elevated liver enzymes.

They discussed the use of milk thistle (for liver support), stress management, education, and therapeutic massage (he was highly stressed). The results in four months were normalized liver enzymes, a greater ability to handle his daily hassles, and he had developed a healthier outlook on life.

You have or will have your own story. You are not alone. Again, if you're not sure, ask about using an alternative or complementary therapy. Be sure to ask; the choices Mary and John made may not be the right ones for you.

GENERAL REMINDERS

Find out the recommended dose for that herb or vitamin or mineral (refer to the resources section). More is not better. Take only what is recommended. Be picky. Ask, ask, and ask again.

Be careful when choosing to take more than one herb at a time or taking a certain herb with specific medications. Don't drink green tea, which has the clotting factor vitamin K, with warfarin, an anticlotting medicine. The effects of this medicine would be lost. It could result in a greater response, such as using large doses of garlic, or *Ginkgo biloba*. If you are taking Coumadin, it may result in unwanted blood thinning.

Specific herbs to avoid, as they can damage the liver, are chaparral, comfrey, germander, jin bu huan, pennyroyal, and poke root. The alert is also out on ephedra (mahuang). It can raise the heart rate and blood pressure. If you're pregnant, don't take anything without the guidance of a health professional. If nursing, consider this same rule. You're feeding the herb not just to yourself but also to another.

Be cautious. Bring your bottles and education sources to the clinic. Buy your herbs from reputable sources. Monitor side effects.

Research

Conventional drugs and treatments are not perfect, but more of them have a known track record. We have only touched the surface in testing alternative and complementary regimens. You may not have the patience to wait. At least read, study, and talk about potential choices before trying them.

Be careful in diagnosing your own symptoms. Many conditions can have the same symptoms. What you choose may not be the best for you because of an inaccurate diagnosis.

Herbs can certainly be an option when you and your physician want to save the use of antibiotics for the specific organisms they are known to treat. Herbs are also useful if the tried and true does not work or along with some other medication to increase the desired response.

Clinical trials are being performed on more herbs to determine their effective use. But just because it is herbal doesn't mean it is safe. Safety should always be the first consideration.

Allopathic health-care providers should not belittle you when you share that you are using certain supplements. Their guidance in using such supplements should be honored. If your health professional does not know about a supplement, ask him or her to find out for you. If you find out, share that information with your health team member.

The relationships among various products when used for a variety of purposes should also be studied. One person was having great difficulty with blood glucose levels until it was found that she was taking a product that had a high sugar content.

Very little is known or recommended about herbal products or supplements for children. Use only with extreme caution.

Also, learn the full name of the herb. Remember the example of lavender. There are many varieties, and one variety is more useful than another for a specific purpose.

Remind yourself that if you have any symptoms within two hours of administration, stop taking that product until you find out otherwise.

American Diabetes Association Guidelines

The American Diabetes Association has specific guidelines for "unproven therapies."

First, they say that unproven therapies have certain characteristics. Too often, the developers don't usually have credentials appropriate to the type of product they're developing. It is possible that they could misinterpret or overrationalize the scientific data in developing or promoting a product. To sell their product they may say it can do more than it actually can. So be a wary buyer.

Second, the American Diabetes Association classifies modalities or products as clearly effective, somewhat effective, unknown or unproven but possibly promising, or clearly ineffective.

You know it is approved for use when given the okay by the Food and Drug Administration (or any other recognized and respected accrediting body).

Look for at least well-controlled studies (studies that compare the group receiving the modality-supplement to a group that gets a placebo or fake pill or another type of treatment) to assure you that the remedy or product is safe. If these well-controlled studies have not been written up in standard, peer-reviewed journals, question the results. You could check with the American Diabetes Association's professional practice committee and see if they endorse or recommend the remedy or product.

Handling Observations

Make notations alongside the notes made for blood glucose testing results or keep a separate diary. Note the time of day a supplement is taken or the modality used and the specific differences it appears to make in your blood glucose readings.

Unless you have kidney or liver problems or both, a week's worth of careful watching will be all that is needed to determine whether a product or therapy has any adverse effects on your body. If you do have kidney or liver problems or both, it would be wise to continue the log and share it with your health professional. The main thing is not to overload damaged liver or kidney functioning. Just as you are asked to decrease your protein intake if you suffer liver or kidney damage, so should extra care be given when taking any supplement.

From a therapeutic standpoint, too much heat or cold could be an added shock the body does not need. Have you experienced being dehydrated in the summertime or getting sunburned? Some remedies that require heat or chemicals could do the same thing, that is, raise your blood sugar.

SOME SUGGESTIONS TO IMPROVE YOUR QUALITY OF LIFE

For improvement of the quality of your life try a combination of two or more of the following:

- humor
- therapeutic massage (including the scalp)
- walking or moving to music
- taking time to breathe deeply
- drinking plenty of fluids (mainly purified water)
- using some aromatherapy
- chewing some sugar-free peppermint gum
- eating plenty of vegetables, fruits, and grains, accompanied with adequate protein
- thinking about or envisioning a peaceful scene

Begin with knowledge. If you have a problem sorting out the information you read, contact a health professional or call the National Center for Complementary and Alternative Medicine clearinghouse (888-644-6226). Determine what self-care behaviors you wish to change. Set up short-term and long-term goals. Start the new behavior in small steps. It is possible that what you change is not for the best. Be willing to revert back to what you were doing before, especially if the change is not working or is giving symptoms that make you feel worse rather than better.

Be sensitive to the way you feel and to the responses noted in your self-monitoring results. Blood glucose monitoring gives you feedback, notably when any change takes place.

CONCLUSION

> "In the end, it's not the years in your life that count,
> it's the life in your years." —*Abraham Lincoln*

There are many therapies and even some supplements that can help you have a brighter, more energetic life. Exploring the use of these is half the fun. If you have never had a therapeutic massage, you're in for a real treat once you find the type of massage you like best. When you develop a program of supplement(s) to be taken at the first symptoms of a cold, and live a life free of upper respiratory infections, that's a blessing, especially if—even with normal blood glucose levels—you have been plagued with frequent illnesses. If you find that using a particular product helps give you more energy in your daily life, along with controlling your blood sugar, then you just feel wonderful.

When someone comes to me, I don't just focus on diabetes and blood sugar records. I want to know how that person sleeps, eats, and handles daily life, besides monitoring the mechanics of the recommended routine and yearly eye exams, yearly physical, and needed laboratory tests.

Problems associated with diabetes management are not just rebalanced by a change in medication, but also by an assessment of lifestyle, pressures, and psychological needs. Questions about your life and the spiritual aspects of daily living also need to be asked. I want to determine if you are using community and religious resources, or is what you need somewhat simple, such as changing a pillow or the choosing a different bedtime snack.

When appropriate, we pray together, use therapeutic touch, or have a healing touch session. I might tell you about Dr. Herbert Benson's relaxation response or give some guidelines on starting a daily meditation practice.

If worse comes to worse, family therapy sessions and stress management counseling is offered. I might ask if you know about a specific herb or remedy that could complement your care. You could then be directed to study such information.

Next, we would discuss the pros and cons. Then you would determine if the herb seemed to be helpful to your particular situation, when and how long you would use it, and what would be the recommended dose and what the side effects might be. If he or she were another physician's patient, the physician would be contacted before the final decision for use was made.

Daily logs would not only include blood glucose results and self-administered medications, but also documentation of the response to the herb. Side effects are asked to be reported promptly.

Become the best detective you can be. Share that information with "the authorities," and work together as a team. You're on the threshold of being even healthier than before. Perhaps what you do in a complementary way will even make it easier to attain and maintain normal blood glucose levels more of the time without experiencing any significant hypoglycemia. What a good feeling that is!

Now that you have more tools, merge that with the knowledge you have about your diabetes management. If you haven't been to a refresher course in diabetes care in the last two years, go to a class so that what you learn in class will be as up-to-date as what you have just learned by reading this book. Combine both types of information and determine what you are going to do to make a better life for yourself and a healthier life for your body.

APPENDIX A

DIABETES: A BRIEF HISTORY OF DIABETES AND TRADITIONAL CARE

by Richard Guthrie, M.D., F.A.C.E., C.D.E.

Diabetes mellitus is a very complex disease. Its treatment is very simple and yet, to others, very complex. When introducing alternative (in place of) and complementary (along with) care, you must have a basic knowledge of the disease, its treatment, and the potential problems that might affect the human body. Therefore this section is meant to give you a background from which you can develop questions to ask yourself or a health professional when you are thinking about using something new in your care that you trust will add years and quality to your life.

Diabetes mellitus (DM) is a group of metabolic diseases characterized by an elevated blood sugar level and its complications, which can be severely disabling and life threatening. The diseases we characterize as DM are ancient. The first description is recorded in an old Egyptian papyrus known as the Ebers Papyrus which dates from the thirteenth century B.C. In this document, a priest described some patients who drank large amounts of fluid and urinated a lot while losing weight. When these people urinated on the ground, the urine attracted ants. It was not until the fifth century A.D. however that the substance attracting the ants was found to be sugar. This was discovered by an Indian physician who found out by tasting the urine and detecting the sweet taste.

In the mid-1800s scientists began to understand the mechanisms of disease for DM. The French physiologist Claude Bernard discovered that when he took the pancreas out of animals they became diabetic. Later the tissue in the pancreas known as the islets of Langerhans was identified as the secretor of a chemical that was responsible for controlling the blood sugar. This substance was called "insuline" or substance of the insular or islet tissue, even though it had not yet been identified. It was not until 1921 that Dr. Fred Banting and Mr. Best, his graduate student, isolated insulin (it lost its *e*) and demonstrated that it controled blood sugar in diabetic animals. In January 1922 they gave the first dose to a human, a boy named Bobby Thompson, in Toronto, Canada, and successfully controlled his blood sugar.

Soon insulin was being extracted from animal pancreases and given to thousands and today millions of people. This discovery was one of the greatest in medical history and has saved millions of lives over the years. But all was not well. It soon became evident that people with diabetes, though kept alive by insulin, went on to develop a variety of chronic complications including blindness, kidney failure, and amputations. More research was needed on how to effectively use this new miracle drug to prevent complications. That research continues to this day.

At the end of World War II, the Germans were experimenting with a group of drugs known as sulfas and found that some of them could be used to bring down blood sugar. This led to the understanding that there was more than one kind of diabetes. There was a form that occurred primarily in children and responded only to insulin, and a form that began primarily in adulthood and could respond at least temporarily to the sulfa pills known as sulfonylureas. In the 1960s the difference between these two forms of diabetes became evident by the discovery of a method of accurately measuring blood insulin levels by Drs. Yalow and Berson. Once they could measure blood insulin levels well, they found that the insulin-dependent people had no internal insulin-producing ability, while the sulfa-responsive people not only could produce insulin, but often had an excessive amount of insulin and were resistant to the action of the insulin produced.

We have subsequently been able to define these diseases much better in recent years, and now know that they are two different diseases, called Type 1 and Type 2 diabetes. Indeed, we know now that there are even different kinds of each of these diseases, so we have many subcategories of the diseases. All are characterized by elevated blood sugar levels and chronic complications, but Type 1 is defined by its insulin deficiency, and Type 2 is defined by its insulin resistance.

Type 1 Diabetes Mellitus (DM)

Type 1 DM is now known to be a disease of the immune system in which, for reasons as yet unknown, the immune system fails and attacks the insulin producing cells of the pancreas and kills them, resulting in insulin deficiency. Without insulin the body cannot get sugar out of the bloodstream and into the cells to be burned. As a result the sugar piles up in the blood while the cells (muscle cells, etc.) are starving. The cells then turn to fat as a source of fuel, and this fat breakdown results in the production of chemicals known as ketones. Ketones can cause the blood to become acidic, which can be fatal. In addition, the body tries to get rid of the excess sugar in the blood by excreting it in the urine. This leads to excess urination (polyuria), since it takes water to get rid of the sugar. The excess urination leads to thirst (polydipsia). The third cardinal sign of Type 1 diabetes is excess hunger (polyphagia) brought about by the fact that the cells are in a state of starvation. In spite of the excess eating the afflicted person loses weight because the food taken in cannot be used for fuel and is subsequently excreted into the urine, enhancing the polyuria and polydipsia. The end result of this sequence of events is diabetic ketoacidosis and death if treatment is not given.

The defect in the immune system that starts the process leading to Type 1 DM is an inherited defect in an immune system gene. Exactly what triggers this gene at a particular time in a person's life is unknown, and while the disease is more common in children, it can come on at any time in life. Some possible triggers that have been studied are viruses, cow's milk, charred food, and chemicals. There are several kinds of Type 1 DM with different triggering agents, but all have in common the destruction of the insulin-producing cells (beta cells) of the pancreas by the immune system resulting in insulin deficiency. Type 1 DM must be treated by insulin injections for the person to live. We may someday find drugs, minerals, herbs, etc., that may mediate the immune process or enhance the action of insulin, but these will be adjuncts (or complementary) and not substitutes for insulin in persons with Type 1 diabetes mellitus.

Type 2 Diabetes Mellitus (DM)

Type 2 DM is the most common form of diabetes, accounting for 90 percent of the some sixteen million people with diabetes in the United States, and is what most people mean when they say they or someone they know has "sugar diabetes." The poor understanding of the difference between Type 1 and Type 2 diabetes often leads to errors in judgment and management. People will hear about a child developing diabetes and say to the parents "Why does your child have to take insulin shots? Why can't he or she take pills like I do?" The answer is they have two different types of diseases that just happen to have similar names. This confusion is often carried over into publications. Many books advocating a variety of alternative medicines and techniques will fail to specify which kind of diabetes they are talking about, and this might give people taking insulin for life a false hope of being able to stop the injections.

Type 2 DM is not a disease of the pancreas initially but rather a condition of insulin resistance by the cells needing insulin such as muscle and fat cells. For some reason insulin does not work right in these individuals and they have to produce more insulin than normal to get the same result. This overwork of the pancreas to produce extra insulin to control the blood sugar and get the sugar into the cells ultimately exhausts the pancreas, which results in a decrease in blood insulin levels and then in an elevated blood sugar. In these individuals the blood insulin levels may still be higher than in a normal person, but it is less than they need, so a relative deficiency results. As in Type 1 diabetes the elevated blood sugar in the cells leads to damage of the blood vessels and nerves and causes the complications of the disease.

Type 2 DM is also an inherited disease, but is inherited differently than Type 1 DM. There are many different kinds of Type 2 DM inherited on different chromosomes and affecting many different places where insulin acts to cause the resistance to its action. In addition to the inheritance factor, there are environmental factors involved in the development of this form of the disease. Type 2 DM is primarily a disease of developed countries, although it is known that peoples all over the world carry the genes for it. So why do we see the disease mainly in developed countries? Because it seems to be associated with the Western lifestyle of excess food intake and decreased energy use, i.e., the sedentary lifestyle of the developed countries. We eat too much and exercise too little and become overweight, which leads to obesity. Somehow obesity leads, in genetically susceptible people, to insulin resistance and later, to diabetes Type 2. We commonly think of this disease as adult onset, and indeed most of it comes on after age forty-five. However, we are seeing it occur earlier and earlier. As our children become fatter and fatter and exercise less and less, we are seeing the beginning of an epidemic of this disease in children. If this is allowed to continue, we face a major problem of diabetes and its complications in the future.

DM Type 2 often has very few symptoms as it is developing. This leads to a delay in diagnosis often for many years. This delay in starting treatment can foster the development of the chronic complications of the disease that are responsible for the horrendous costs of the disease to our society. The current estimate of the cost of diabetes in the United States is $138 billion per year. About $100 billion dollars of that is spent on treatment for the complications of the disease, a situation made more tragic by the fact that most of the complications of diabetes are preventable if the disease is diagnosed early and treated adequately. The diagnosis is made on the basis of a fasting plasma glucose (FPG) of 126 mg/dL (7 mmol/L) or greater, or a random plasma glucose level of greater than 200 (11.1 mmol/L) if symptoms are present, or a value at two hours, after a specific amount of glucose is given, of 200 (11.1 mmol/L) or greater. Values less than these but greater than normal are called impaired fasting glucose (IFG) (110 [6.5 mmol/L] to 125 mg/dL [6.9 mmol/L]) or impaired glucose tolerance (IGT). The old term used for these latter groups—borderline diabetes—should no longer be used.

Type 2 diabetes is a very complex group of diseases, and it is important to understand the way the body works in order to understand where each of the medicines fits into the treatment scheme. The treatment is different, for example, if the problem is primarily insulin resistance rather than a nonworking pancreas and insulin deficiency (few beta cells working if at all). It would make no sense to give a drug that stimulates insulin secretion if the problem is insulin resistance. Likewise, if the problem is insulin deficiency, giving only an insulin sensitizer would not work well. So if we understand that the initial problem is insulin resistance and later insulin deficiency, we can plug in the appropriate treatments at the proper times.

TREATMENT OF DIABETES MELLITUS

Type 2 Diabetes

Diet, Exercise, Lifestyle Change, and Drug Therapy.   If the fasting plasma glucose (FPS) is above 126 mg/dL (7 mmol/L) but less than 200 mg/dL (11.1 mmol/L), treatment can be initiated by education in diet, exercise, and lifestyle change. Mild elevation of the FPS indicates insulin resistance without damage as yet to the insulin-producing cells of the pancreas (beta cells). If we then can relieve the cause of the insulin resistance, i.e., overeating, underexercising, and obesity, then we should be able to return the blood sugar to normal. But all these individuals should be trained in self-monitoring of blood glucose (SMBG), and should have intensive dietary training and be given a structured exercise program or guided into a lifestyle that includes increased physical activity. This training is not different no matter the type or severity of the diabetes. Diet, exercise, and SMBG are keys to good diabetes control and will be discussed in more detail later.

When the FPS is above 200 mg/dL (11.1 mmol/L) but less than 300 mg/dL (16.6 mmol/L), therapy should be initiated with an oral antidiabetic drug in addition to diet and exercise. Likewise if the initial therapy of diet and exercise does not work (FPS remains above 126 mg/dL [7 mmol/L] or hemoglobin A_{1c} remains above 8 percent) then oral medication should be added. There are several oral medications that can be used:

A. First generation agents
   1. tolbutamide (Orinase)
   2. tolazamide (Tolinase)
   3. acetohexamide (Dymelar)
   4. chlorpropamide (Diabinese)

B. Second generation agents
   1. glyburide (Micronase, DiaBeta, and Glynase)
   2. glipizide (Glucotrol and Glucotrol XL)
   3. glimiperide (Amaryl)

C. metformin (Glucophage)
D. acarbose (Precose); miglitol (Glyset)
E. troglitazone (Rezulin); rosiglitazone (Avandia); pioglitazone (Actos)
F. repaglinide (Prandin)

First generation oral agents are no longer used so will not be discussed here. Second generation sulfonylurea agents have been available for over ten years and continue in widespread use. There is little difference among the agents except in dose and time action, with Amaryl and Glucotrol XL being the longest acting; they are usually once-a-day drugs, which makes them more convenient to take. All of these drugs work in essentially the same way. They stimulate the beta cells of the pancreas to produce more insulin. Thus they are useful in the moderately severe diabetes states where there is decreased insulin production and insulin resistance. These drugs are usually given once or twice a day and usually before meals. They are usually effective in controlling blood sugar, if combined with diet and exercise and weight loss, for a period of three to ten years with an average duration of use of five years.

The next drug to be introduced to the United States was metformin (Glucophage). This drug had been used in most of the world for over twenty years before it became available in the United States. It has now been available over five years. This drug works entirely differently from the sulfonyurea drugs. This drug works primarily in the liver to suppress production of sugar by the liver. It also works to increase use of sugar by the muscle cells, all of which reduces the sugar in the blood. The primary side effect of this drug is upset stomach and diarrhea, both of which are usually short-lived (two weeks or less). This drug can also produce a state called lactic acidosis, which is highly fatal. Lactic acid in the bloodstream can lead to death if this acid can't be processed by the liver and/or released from the body through functioning kidneys. Therefore, metformin should never be given to anyone who has other diseases that may support the development of lactic acidosis (kidney or liver disease, severe infection especially of the lungs, asthma, heart failure, etc.), and any time an iodine-containing dye is to be used (intravenous pylogram, heart catheterization, angiogram, etc.). The drug is useful as a single agent or in combination with any of the other agents or insulin. The starting dose is 500 mg (one pill) with breakfast or supper. The dose can be increased to a maximum dose of 2,500 mg (five pills per day, or three 850-mg pills per day, or two 1,000-mg pills and one 500-mg pill per day distributed throughout the day with meals).

Acarbose was the next drug introduced in the United States. It also had been used for many years in other parts of the world. This drug works by preventing the breakdown and absorption of starch in the bowel. Normally starch (like potatoes or pasta, etc.) are digested in the upper part of the intestinal tract from long chains of sugars to individual sugars, and then absorbed. It is this breakdown that is blocked so the sugars cannot be absorbed and cannot therefore raise the blood sugar. The major side effect of this agent is intestinal gas. When the starch is not digested in the upper tract, it passes to the lower intestinal tract, where it is acted on by the bacteria found there and fermented into gas. This drug is useful in diabetes treatment when people are having problems keeping the after-meal blood sugars down but has not been popular in the United States because of the flatulence (gas formation). The drug is given with the first bite of food at each meal starting with a low dose (25 mg/one time a day) and raising the dose as tolerance to the side effects occurs (to a total of 50 mg three times a day for those weighing 132 lbs or less and 100 mg three times a day for those weighing over 132 lbs). A more recently released pill, Glyset, at the 50-mg dose, taken with each meal, is reported to result in less gas formation.

Troglitazone or Rezulin (a first generation drug) is a drug belonging to an entirely new class of drugs recently discovered. This drug and others in its (second generation) class (such as rosiglitazone [Avandia] or pioglitazone [Actos]) work by stimulating a gene in the cell nucleus that causes the production of a chemical called a glucose transporter. These chemicals, produced inside the cell, migrate to the cell surface and "suck" the sugar and other larger molecular substances such as protein into the cell, thus reducing the blood sugar level. It has very few side effects. But Rezulin has led to damage of the liver, and has been fatal for some (0.02 percent of the total number taking the medication). It is vital that the doctor monitor the liver enzymes monthly, and, for Actos and Avandia, for the first year of therapy every two months and then routinely. The liver damage is reversible if detected early and the drug stopped. The major disadvantage of this drug is its slow onset of action. It can take as long as six to twelve weeks to have its optimal effect, and rarely will it have any effect for the first two to four weeks. Thus it is not a good agent to initiate therapy in a newly diagnosed person with a 300 mg/dL (16.6 mmol/L) or higher blood sugar, but is better used in combination with other drugs for later therapy. The initial dose of Rezulin is 200 mg once a day with food (which enhances its absorption). The dose can be increased to a maximum dose of 600 mg per day. This drug has been very effective in controlling blood sugar, especially when combined with other drugs. Rosiglitazone (Avandia), a second generation drug having lower dosage levels, has little if any effect on the liver (initial dose of 2 or 4 mg with a maximum dose of 8 mg). Pioglitazone (Actos): initial dose of 15 or 30 mg with a maximum dose of 45 mg/day.

Repaglinide (Prandin) is a new drug that works like the sulfonylurea drugs to stimulate insulin release, but it is not a sulfonylurea. It is a derivative of benzoic acid. It differs from the sulfonylureas in that it is very short-acting. It is given with or within fifteen minutes of the meal, acts quickly to keep down postmeal blood sugar, and is gone in about three hours. Thus it is very helpful for those who have aftermeal elevated blood sugar, and its short effect doesn't last to cause low blood sugar later. It is less helpful when the fasting sugar in the morning is elevated. The side effects are the same as the sulfonylureas, that is, mostly low blood sugar if the dose is too high. The starting dose is 0.5 mg with each meal and can be increased to a maximum dose of 4 mg with each meal and bedtime snack (a total maximum dose of 16 mg per day).

In Type 2 diabetes these drugs can be used alone or in combination. Usually they are started alone—called monotherapy. If monotherapy will not control the blood sugar or the glycated hemoglobin (HbA$_{1c}$), then a second drug is added, or even a third, as they can complement one another through different mechanisms of action. The sulfonylureas and repaglinides work by stimulating insulin production while metformin and troglitazone work to make the insulin work better, that is, reduce insulin resistance, and acarbose and precose work to prevent the absorption of sugar in the first place. All of the drugs can be used with insulin, or insulin alone may be used in people with Type 2 diabetes when the oral agents are no longer effective.

Type 1 Diabetes

Since Type 1 diabetes is caused by insulin deficiency, treatment can only be by insulin replacement, which must be given by injection. There are several kinds of insulin we can use to replace that which is missing. What we must do in the treatment of Type 1 diabetes is to simulate what the body normally does in insulin production. The way the normal body works is to produce a small amount of insulin all the time, every day. This is called basal insulin. Then the body secretes a burst or bolus of insulin to increase blood insulin levels when we eat to handle the food (first-stage insulin release) and then secretes another burst about an hour and a half later (second-stage insulin release). The closer we can simulate this action the better control we will have. We must therefore understand the kinds of insulin we have and how to use them to this end.

1. Very short-acting insulin (very rapid-acting insulin). This is the newest type of insulin on the market. It is called an insulin ana-logue or designer insulin, i.e., the sequence of two amino acids in the chemical insulin chain have been switched around. The name of this first rapid-acting insulin is lispro or Humalog insulin. Like all insulin, it is now made synthetically. A single change in one of the two normal human insulin chains gives it its very rapid action. This insulin has its onset of action five to fifteen minutes after injection, reaches its peak effect in one to two hours and is gone in three to four hours. It is taken right before the meal and has its peak effect at the same time the food is being maximally absorbed. Thus it matches to food much better than other insulin and is therefore more conducive to the fast lifestyle that most of us lead. However, it must be combined with a longer acting insulin for nighttime and sometimes daytime coverage.

2. Short-acting insulin—regular insulin (crystalline insulin or Act-rapid insulin). This insulin is identical to the insulin produced in the pan-creas by normal people but acts somewhat differently when given by injection under the skin. The onset of action is thirty to sixty min-utes, a peak effect is achieved in two to three hours, and has an ef-fective therapeutic or pharmacodynamic duration of action of four to six hours (the pharmacokinetic action of insulin, or zero insulin

levels to zero insulin levels, is two to five hours at the peak and five to eight hours for the duration). It must be taken thirty or more minutes before a meal in order to have an effect on the food eaten one hour later. Failure to do this is a common cause of poor diabetes control. In addition, this insulin can last until the next meal and may cause premeal hypoglycemia or low blood sugar. It is not the ideal insulin for our busy lives, but until lispro insulin became available it was the best we had. The majority of people taking insulin use it.

3. Intermediate-acting insulin. There are two insulins in this group— NPH (Neutral Protamine Hagedorn—Dr. Hagedorn was the man who first developed this insulin) and Lente insulin. These insulins have an onset of action (therapeutically) of about one to a little over two hours after injection, a peak effect in six to eight hours, and last from twelve to sixteen hours (therapeutically) and peak in six to twelve hours and last sixteen to twenty-four hours (chemically, or zero to zero insulin levels). They are most useful as a background insulin used twice a day to provide the basal insulin need, but they do little to provide the bolus effect (rapid effect) with meals. These insulins are rarely used alone, unless used at bedtime. They are usually prescribed in combination with short-acting or rapid-acting insulin, which is given with meals against the foundation of NPH or Lente. Lente has a slightly longer peak and duration of action when compared to NPH.

4. Long-acting insulin. We currently have only one insulin in this class—Ultralente. This insulin has its onset of action in about two to four hours after injection, its peak effect comes in eight to fifteen hours and a duration of effect of eighteen to twenty-four hours (pharmacokinetically, peaks in eight to twenty hours and has a duration of twenty-four to twenty-eight hours). This insulin is used exclusively for a background or basal insulin. It can be given once or twice a day but always must be combined with a very rapid- or short-acting insulin for meal boluses.

Knowing the need for basal and bolus insulin and the time action of the various insulins, we can then develop an almost infinite number of ways to combine them to meet the needs of almost everyone. The common methods of management are listed below:

1. Four to five doses per day of regular insulin. This is primarily a hospital-based regimen, since many people do not like to take four or more injections per day or to stay up until midnight or later to take the last injection. Its use in the hospital and sometimes on an

outpatient basis is to attain control of the blood sugar in a person whose sugar is out of control. A total daily dose of insulin is calculated, based on previous dosage or on body weight, and is given as regular insulin: 35 percent for breakfast, 22 percent for lunch, 28 percent for supper, and 15 percent at midnight. Doses are then adjusted based on the previous day's blood sugar values. Multiple injections lead to increased flexibility of lifestyle and potential for more normal blood sugars more of the time.

2. Three or four injections per day of regular and NPH or Lente insulin. If four or five doses of insulin per day are needed but the person does not want to stay up until midnight, an intermediate-acting insulin can be given at bedtime and the regular (crystalline or Actrapid) or lispro insulin given with meals.

3. Three injections per day. Many regimens use three injections per day. Regular (short-acting) or lispro (rapid-acting) can be given with meals and NPH or Lente at supper time. Ultralente can be given once or twice a day with regular or lispro at meals, or a mixture of regular or lispro with NPH or Lente at breakfast, regular or lispro at supper and NPH or Lente at bedtime. Other regimens are possible, but the above are the most commonly used three-dose methods.

4. Two doses per day. To achieve twenty-four-hour basal and meal bolus insulin with only two doses of insulin per day a mixture of regular or lispro and NPH or Lente must be given with breakfast and supper. This regimen is commonly used but is only moderately effective and usually cannot be used for very long if good control is to be maintained. This regimen is now known as conventional therapy, while more than two injections a day of insulin is known as intensive therapy.

General Treatment of Type 1 and 2 Diabetes Mellitus

Nutrition.   There are many forms of nutritional therapy recommended for people with diabetes. The most common today are the exchange list (six food groupings), the point system (one point equals seventy-five calories), and carbohydrate (CHO) counting (15 gms per count). Each system has good and bad points, but nutritional control is vital to diabetes control. The meal plan should not be viewed as difficult or burdensome. It is nothing more or less than a healthful well-balanced diet anyone wanting to remain in good health should eat. The diet consists of healthful meals rich in fruits and vegetables, a moderate amount of protein, a liberal amount of complex carbohydrates (grains, lentils), a low fat content, and a good fiber and fluid intake.

The meal plan for the person who has diabetes is similar to the prudent American diet recommended by the American Heart Association for good heart health. Calories should be appropriate for growth in children and for attaining and maintaining proper weight in adults. Food should be eaten in similar amounts throughout the day, and should usually include a bedtime snack. Large infrequent meals should be avoided, as it is difficult to match the insulin or pills to these large meals and attempts to do so can lead to obesity. What system of diet one uses is less important than to remember the biblical admonition to "be moderate in all things." The system used is just a tool to help remember to choose the right foods at the right times.

Exercise.   In modern-day society with its myriad of machines to do our work for us, we get very little physical activity. Our ancestors, who had to walk long distances, follow the horse in the furrow while guiding the plow, wash clothes on a washboard, beat rugs over the line, and chop and carry wood to the stove burned from three to five thousand calories per day. We in the modern age ride in cars, take elevators, do work by machines in the home and office and therefore burn less than two thousand calories per day. Yet most of us want to eat like our ancestors, and consume more than three thousand calories per day. If we are to do so, we must devise ways to expend that extra one thousand calories or we will get fat fast. Taking in two hundred calories a day (equal to two and a half slices of bread) more than we burn up can result in gaining a pound every two weeks or twenty-six pounds a year. We must therefore decrease our intake or devise exercise programs to burn the calories. There is no alternative and no "magic bullet."

One of the best forms of exercise is walking. Running brings no added benefit to weight control. Walking or running for two miles burns the same number of calories. Running will, however, get you finished faster and is better at toning the heart and muscles, but it offers no advantage for calorie burning or obesity control. Everyone should walk two miles a day or more or do some exercise (swimming, cycling, etc.) every day. Devising some form of exercise is vital but should be something you enjoy so that you can stay with it. The exercise should also be matched with the medicine prescribed and the meals consumed so that hypoglycemia does not occur. It is not a good idea, for example, to get up in the morning, take your insulin, and go for a two-mile walk before you eat breakfast. Walk after breakfast or delay your insulin until you return. Use common sense and you will do well.

Monitoring.   If you were traveling to a strange place, you would want to have a map or one of those new global locators in order to know where you are. Think of monitoring your blood sugar as your map that tells you where you are and what you need to do to get where you want to go to obtain the best diabetes control you can achieve for a long and healthy life. Self-monitoring is necessary for every person with diabetes, no matter what kind they have or what the treatment program. Monitoring is done by sticking the body and obtaining a small drop of blood that is then put on a strip of paper that contains a chemical that reacts with the sugar in the blood, causing a color change in the strip or generates an electrical charge, either of which can then be read in a small handheld machine. These machines are small, inexpensive, and give a rapid (in seconds) and accurate readout of the blood sugar. Newly diagnosed persons with diabetes and those whose sugars are out of control should test a minimum of four times a day every day until control is established. If blood sugars are good and the medicine dose is stable for a few weeks, you can decrease the testing to four times a day three to four days a week. People on diet therapy alone can get by with testing four times a day one to two days a week. You should never test fewer than four times per day on the day you test because you need to determine how your body responds to the medication in relation to your food and activity/or illness response. If on very rapid-acting insulin or rapid-acting oral agent (repaglinide), testing before breakfast and two hours after a meal gives you more information than just the usual premeal and bedtime blood sugar, because blood sugar is not the same at different times of the day especially for those on medication. Never cheat or skimp on blood sugar monitoring. This is your lifeline to a longer, healthier, and more productive life.

Stress Management.   Stress is a constant of modern-day life. As life gets faster and more complicated, our stress levels go up. Stress can have a detrimental effect on blood sugar. During times of stress, the body produces hormones such as adrenaline (epinephrine) and cortisone, which raise blood sugar and throw off control. It is therefore imperative that we learn ways to cope with stress so our hormones can return to normal and let the blood sugar settle down. There are many ways to cope and many of these have been dealt with in this book. Read them and practice them so they can be useful to you in handling the many stresses of life we all must face. We all must make choices in life. The trick is to make the choices that simplify rather than complicate.

Sometimes we have no control over the stresses and in that case we must develop coping skills and relaxing exercises that will restore tranquillity. Those who learn these skills will do well and will be able to attain and maintain control of their diabetes and their lives.

COMPLICATIONS

The primary cost of diabetes comes not in the hassles of daily care, but in the short- and long-term complications of the disease. Short-term complications are hypoglycemia and diabetic ketoacidosis. Long-term complications include large vessel disease, small vessel disease, and neurologic disease.

Short-Term Complications

Hypoglycemia or low blood sugar results in shakiness, sweating, palpitations of the heart, hunger, blurring of vision, inappropriate behavior, and eventually coma and convulsions. The loss of control that occurs with the latter symptoms can result in injury and death. Prolonged, severe, recurrent hypoglycemia can result in permanent brain damage.

Hypoglycemia is seen primarily in people with Type 1 diabetes, but can occasionally be seen in people with Type 2 diabetes if they have kidney disease or are overdosed on the oral hypoglycemic medications or insulin. The cause of hypoglycemia can be due to overdose of medications, improper timing of medications, food or exercise, undereating, or overexercising. The problem may be the result of patient error or the wrong regimen for that person's lifestyle. An example of the latter is the use of high doses of long-acting insulin given too frequently, such as NPH insulin three or more times a day. The cause of the hypoglycemia must be searched for and corrected for the safety of the individual.

Treatment of hypoglycemia is with food (if recognized early on) or glucose administered quickly by a route appropriate to the degree of impairment. If the treatment is given early enough, while the person experiencing moderate (blood sugar levels in the forties or less) hypoglycemia is coherent, then glucose or sugar may be given by mouth. There are commercial forms of glucose available, or table sugar may be given in some palatable form such as candy, soft drink, or juice. This should be followed with solid food after recovery (usually ten to fifteen minutes later). In the case of deeper loss of control, the commercial glucose products, such as Glutose or Monogel, or honey may be placed in the cheek or under the tongue. When coma or seizure occurs something must be given by a route other than by mouth, since substances in the mouth may be aspirated into the lung with resulting pneumonia. A substance called glucagon should be available at all times to be injected in the vein, under the skin, or in the muscle. When medical personnel are available the concentrated 10 to 50 percent glucose should be injected in the vein.

Diabetic Ketoacidosis (DKA).   DKA is seen only in Type 1 diabetes or in someone whose Type 2 diabetes has regressed to a point of no beta cell function, and is the result of inadequate amounts of available insulin. This can be due to being a new diabetic not yet treated, to missing insulin doses, or to an increased need, such as during infection or treatment with certain medications such as steroids.

Symptoms of DKA are increased urination, thirst and hunger with weight loss, rapid respiration, dehydration, rapid pulse, low blood pressure, and eventually coma and death if untreated. Signs of DKA are a concentrated urine with ketones, elevated blood sugar, and dry skin and membranes. In the most severe state there can be abdomen or chest pain, coma, shock, and imbalance of the blood chemistries with high sugar, low salts, and low carbon dioxide in the blood.

Treatment of this condition is rapid rehydration with fluids and the addition of salts and intravenous insulin.

Long-Term Complications

Large Vessel Disease (LVD)   in diabetes is no different from LVD in the nondiabetic except that it can occur at an earlier age and can affect young women as well as men. The lesions seen are the same as in other people, such as atherosclerosis, with lesions in the arteries of the heart, neck, and cerebral vessels and in the legs. In the person with diabetes, these lesions look the same and the effects are the same (heart attacks, strokes, blockages in the legs, etc.) but they can occur much earlier. Men and women in their twenties can develop these lesions and their consequences. Chest pain in a twenty-five-year-old woman without diabetes is not likely to be heart related, but the same pain in a similar woman with more than ten years of diabetes is very likely to be cardiac. Symptoms in LVD in diabetes are the same as in the nondiabetic.

Similarly, treatment is the same as in the nondiabetic and will not be further discussed here. However, more important is the prevention of these lesions by diet, exercise, control of cholesterol and triglycerides, and tight control of blood sugar. There is now good evidence that high blood sugar is a significant contributor to the development of LVD and must be controlled: this means following a good diet, exercising regularly, and controlling blood sugar by proper medication, and daily blood sugar monitoring, as well as having frequent medical checkups with measurements of sugar, lipids, blood pressure, and hemoglobin A_{1c} (Hgb A_{1c}).

Small Vessel Disease (microvascular disease—MVD).   Involves the small blood vessels (capillaries) all over the body and is specific to diabetes. The disease is manifest primarily in the eye and the kidney, resulting in possible blindness and kidney failure. The lesions found in these organs are similar and involve thickening (by separation of layers of the walls of the blood vessels) and thereby weakening of the capillary walls with compromise of the lumen or interior of the vessel and breakage with hemorrhage. This can result in inadequate blood flow to the important parts of the eye and kidney needed for their proper function. The result of this damage is blindness and kidney failure. Diabetes is the leading cause of adult blindness and the leading cause of kidney dialysis and transplant and is a major cause of the cost of diabetes both in money and in human suffering.

The cause of these lesions is now being understood. The cells that line the blood vessels of the eye and kidney, unlike other tissues, are permeable to sugar without the help of insulin. So the level of sugar (glucose) inside the cell will be the same as the level of sugar in the lumen of the blood vessel. But how levels of sugar in excess of about 120 mg/dL (6.1 mmol/L) are toxic to these cells and how they become damaged by several mechanisms is now being worked out by scientists around the world. Suffice it to say here, the excess sugar attaches to parts of the cells and interferes with their normal action and may even kill the cells. This then prevents the normal flow of blood to the organs such as the eye and kidney, which these vessels serve, causing damage to the organ. What this tells us is that we can prevent these lesions and the subsequent organ damage by keeping the blood sugar down at normal levels as much of the time as possible.

The lesions can be treated if they are "allowed" to occur, but prevention is the better choice. Treatment of the eye lesions is by laser surgery and by inter-eye surgery to reattach the retina when it detaches. Treatment of the kidney consists of a low-protein diet, meticulous blood pressure control usually with a drug of the class called ACE inhibitors (angiotension converting enzymes), and control of blood sugar.

When the kidney deteriorates to the point where it is essentially nonfunctional, then there are two courses of action—dialysis (filtering the waste products of the blood by circulating it from the body into the filtering machine, and then back to the body) or transplant. Both of these procedures are expensive and not wholly satisfactory. Prevention by control of blood sugar and blood pressure is much cheaper and much more satisfactory.

Neuropathy.   This is a common complication of both Type 1 and Type 2 diabetes and develops very early in the course of the disease. The process of nerve damage usually begins in the feet and moves upward. The usual presenting symptoms are pain, burning, and tingling followed by numbness (or polyneuropathy). The motor nerves can also be involved with wasting of the muscles and weakness of the muscles of the feet, legs, and later the arms. These problems are caused by hooking sugar onto the nerve cells in much the same way that the blood vessels are damaged and is therefore caused by high blood sugar, and these problems are therefore preventable. The consequence of the nerve damage is pain, numbness, foot ulcers, muscle weakness, inability to walk, etc. The internal nervous system can also be involved with resulting problems such as gastroparesis (paralysis of the stomach) with vomiting and starvation, diarrhea (especially at night), low blood pressure on standing (can be accompanied by fainting on standing), bladder paralysis with incontinence and urinary tract infection, erectile dysfunction, and others. These lesions are very disabling, can be fatal, and must be prevented. (Mononeuopathy—or one-sided neuropathy—is usually not associated with blood sugar control.)

Treatment of these lesions is most unsatisfactory. Pain medications are only marginally effective and often must be given in such doses as to be toxic or addicting. There are other medications that can be used, but all of them are potent and cause many side effects and are often not very effective. Prevention is the important issue in neuropathy and is accomplished by tight control of the blood sugar. Early lesions are reversible with tight control of the blood sugar.

SUMMARY

Diabetes mellitus in its various forms is a common disease and is becoming more common every day. It is a disabling and costly disease in both money and human suffering. With our present knowledge the disease is not preventable, but it may be in the future. The disease is not curable but it is treatable. New methods of treatment and monitoring have been developed in recent years, and the march forward continues. The most serious problem with the disease is not in the day-to-day care of the disease but the complications. The tragedy of these complications is that most are preventable by known methods of control available today. Many people are not now receiving this care for a variety of reasons and many are not complying with the treatment available, so that the complications continue to be a source of monetary loss and human disability and suffering. The future is bright, however, if we continue our efforts at research and treatment and avail ourselves of as much education as possible about the disease and every treatment modality that can be developed. There have been in the past, however, many inappropriate treatments that have been harmful or at best ineffective thus depriving the person with diabetes of the preventative care they need. We should look at all possible treatments and miss none that have proven effective, but we should remember that all modes of treatment or prevention must be subjected to the most careful research and trial to prove not only effectiveness but safety as well. A cardinal rule of medicine since the time of Hippocrates is "first do no harm." It must be our axiom today as well.

Appendix B

Vitamins and Minerals

Summary: Fat-Soluble Vitamins

Vitamin*		Function	Deficiency	Sources
A (Retinol—precursor carotenes)		Formation of visual purple; normal growth of epithelial tissue, especially skin and mucous membranes; normal bone and tooth structure.	Night and glare blindness; deterioration of epithelial tissue leading to decreased resistance to infection; dry scaly skin; eye changes; xerophthalmia leading to blindness	Liver, whole milk, and foods containing milk fat such as butter, cream, cheese, margarine; as carotene in dark green leafy vegetables, carrots, and some fruits
RDI:				
Birth–1 Year	375 mcg (125 IU)			
1–3 Years	400 mcg (133 IU)			
4–6 Years	500 mcg (166 IU)			
7–10 Years.	700 mcg (233 IU)			
11 Years to Adult:				
Females	800 mcg (266 IU)			
Males	1,000 mcg (333 IU)			
D (Calciferol)		Promotion of absorption of calcium and phosphorus; normal utilization of these minerals in skeleton and soft tissue.	Faulty bone and tooth development; rickets; osteomalacia	Fortified milk; direct exposure of skin to sunlight; fish, liver oils
RDI:				
Birth–6 months	7.5 mcg (300 IU)			
6 months—18 years	10 mcg (400 IU)			

*Recommended Dietary Allowances (RDA)

(continued)

Summary: Fat-Soluble Vitamins *(continued)*

Vitamin	Function	Deficiency	Sources
E (Tocopherols) RDI: Birth–1 Year 3–4 mg (3–4 IU) 1–3 Years 6 mg (6 IU) 4–10 Years 7 mg (7 IU) 11 Years to Adult Females 8 mg (8 IU) Males 10 mg (10 IU)	Antioxidation—protection of substances that oxidize readily, such as vitamin A and essential fatty acids; thus, prevention of damage to cell membranes	Destruction of red blood cells (hemolysis); deficiency is rare	Vegetable oils and shortening; margarine; green leafy vegetables; whole grains; legumes, nuts
K (Menadione) Birth –1 Year 5–10 mcg 1–3 Years 15 mcg 4–6 Years 20 mcg 7–10 Years 30 mcg 11–14 Years 45 mcg 15–18 Years Females 55 mcg Males 65 mcg	Normal blood clotting	Prolonged clotting time; hemorrhagic disease in newborns	Synthesis by intestinal bacteria; green leafy vegetables

Summary: Fat-Soluble Vitamins (*continued*)

Vitamin		Function	Deficiency	Sources
C (Ascorbic Acid)		Collagen formation: strong blood vessels, healthy skin, healthy gums, wound healing; formation of red blood cells: absorption of iron, conversion of folacin to its active form	Adult acne; easy bruising; poor wound healing; swanneck hair deformity; sore gums: hemorrhages around bones; scurvy	Citrus fruit; broccoli, strawberries; cantaloupe, guava, mango, papaya; peppers; green tomatoes; potatoes
RDI:				
Birth–1 Year	30–35 mg			
1–3 Years	40 mg			
4–10 Years	45mg			
11–14 Years	50 mg			
15–18 Years	60 mg			
B₁ (Thiamin)		Energy metabolism; synthesis of DNA, RNA	Poor appetite; fatigue; constipation; neuritis of legs: beriberi; wasting paralysis of legs; heart failure; mental confusion	Meats, especially pork; wheat germ; whole-grain and enriched bread; legumes; peanuts, peanut butter; nuts
RDI:				
Birth–1 Year	0.3–0.4 mg			
1–3 Years	0.7 mg			
4–6 Years	0.9 mg			
7–10 Years	1 mg			
11–14 Years				
Females	1.1 mg			
Males	1.3 mg			
15–18 Years				
Females	1.1 mg			
Males	1.5 mg			

(*continued*)

Summary: Fat-Soluble Vitamins (*continued*)

Vitamin	Function	Deficiency	Sources
B$_2$ (Riboflavin) RDI:	Energy metabolism; protein metabolism	Sensitivity to light; eye irritation; cheilosis; glossitis	Milk; organ meats; meat, fish, eggs; green leafy vegetables; enriched breads and cereals
Birth–1 Year 0.4–0.5 mg			
1–3 Years 0.8 mg			
4–6 Years 1.1 mg			
7–10 Years 1.2 mg			
11–14 Years			
Females 1.3mg			
Males 1.5 mg			
15–18 Years			
Females 1.3 mg			
Males 1.8 mg			
B$_3$ (Niacin) RDI:	Energy metabolism; production fatty acids, cholesterol, steroid hormones	Fatigue; poor appetite; weakness; anxiety; pellagra; diarrhea, dermatitis, deteriorated mental state	Liver, meat, fish, poultry; peanuts; legumes; whole-grain breads and cereals; sources of tryptophan: complete protein foods
Birth–1 Year 5–6 mg			
1–3 Years 9 mg			
4–6 Years 12 mg			
7–10 Years 13 mg			
11–14 Years			
Females 15 mg			
Males 17 mg			
15–18 Years			
Females 1.5 mg			
Males 20 mg			

Summary: Fat-Soluble Vitamins (*continued*)

Vitamin		Function	Deficiency	Sources
B$_6$ (Pyridoxine) RDI:		Amino acid metabolism involving protein synthesis; synthesis of regulatory substances such as serotonin; niacin production; hemoglobin synthesis	Anemia; sore mouth; nausea; dermatities; irritability; convulsions	Liver, kidney, red meats; corn; whole-grain cereals; legumes; bananas; potatoes; green vegetables
Birth–1 Year	0.3–0.6 mg			
1–3 Years	1 mg			
4–6 Years	1.1 mg			
7–10 Years	1.4 mg			
11–14 Years				
Females	1.4 mg			
Males	1.7 mg			
15–18 Years				
Females	1.5 mg			
Males	2 mg			
B$_8$ (Pantothenic acid)		Energy metabolism; synthesis of amino acids, fatty acids, cholesterol, steroid hormones, hemoglobin	Unlikely unless part of a deficiency of all B vitamins	Organ meats; salmon; eggs; broccoli; mushrooms; pork; whole grains; legumes; (synthesized by intestinal bacteria)

(*continued*)

Summary: Fat-Soluble Vitamins (*continued*)

Vitamin	Function	Deficiency	Sources
B₁₂ (Cobalamin)	Protein metabolism; synthesis of DNA, production of red blood cells; healthy nervous system; carbohydrate metabolism, myelin formation (intrinsic factor of gastric secretions is required for absorption)	Pernicious anemia; macrocytic anemia, sore mouth, poor appetite, poor coordination in walking, mental disturbances	Found only in animal products; meat, fish, poultry, eggs, milk, cheese
RDI:			
Birth–1 Year 0.3–0.5 mcg			
1–3 Years 0.7 mcg			
4–6 Years 1 mcg			
7–10 Years 1.4 mcg			
11–Adult 2 mcg			
Folic acid (Folacin)	Protein metabolism; synthesis of DNA and RNA, red blood cell formation	Macrocytic anemia	Green leafy vegetables; liver, kidney, meats, fish; nuts; legumes; whole grains
RDI:			
Birth–1 Year 25–35 mg			
1–3 Years 50 mg			
4–6 Years 75 mg			
7–10 Years 100 mg			
11–14 Years 150 mg			
15–18 Years			
Females 180 mg			
Males 200 mg			

Summary: Minerals

Mineral	Function	Deficiency	Sources
Calcium	Bone and tooth formation; blood clotting; cell permeability; nerve stimulation; muscle contraction; enzyme activation	Stunted growth, rickets, osteomalacia; osteoporosis (porous bones); tetany (low serum calcium)	Milk, hard boiled eggs and small fish eaten with bones; some dark green vegetables; legumes
Chromium	Possibly improve insulin sensitivity and decrease triglyceride levels	Increase imunoreaction insulin	Whole grains, bran, egg yolks, liver and brewer's yeast
Fluorine	Resists dental decay	Tooth decay in young children	Fluoridated water (1 ppm*)
Iodine	Synthesis of thyroid hormones that regulate basal metabolic rate	Goiter, cretinism, if deficiency is severe	Iodized salt; seafood; food grown near the sea
Iron	Hemoglobin and myoglobin formation; cellular enzymes	Anemia	Liver, lean meats, legumes, dried fruits, green leafy vegetables; whole-grain and fortified cereals
Magnesium	Component of bones and teeth; activates any enzymes, including those involved in energy metabolism; nerve stimulation; muscle contraction	Seen in alcoholism or renal disease; tremors leading to convulsive seizures	Green leafy vegetables; nuts, whole grains; meat; milk; seafood

*ppm = parts per million

(continued)

Summary: Minerals (*continued*)

Mineral	Function	Deficiency	Sources
Phosphorus	Bone and tooth formation; energy metabolism—component of DNA and RNA; fat transport; acid-base balance; enzyme formation	Stunted growth; rickets (due to excessive excretion rather than to dietary deficiency)	Distributed widely in foods; milk; meats, poultry, fish, eggs; cheese; nuts; legumes; whole grains; processed foods
Sodium	Osmotic pressure; water balance; acid-base balance; nerve stimulation; muscle contraction; cell permeability	Rare; nausea; vomiting; giddiness; exhaustion; cramps	Table salt, salted foods, MSG and other sodium additives; milk; meat, fish, poultry, eggs
Potassium	Osmotic pressure; water balance; acid-base balance; nerve stimulation; muscle contraction; synthesis of protein; glycogen formation	Nausea; vomiting; muscular weakness; rapid heartbeat; heart failure	Widely distributed in food, meats, fish, poultry; whole grains; fruits, vegetables, legumes
Zinc	Constituent of many enzyme systems, including those involved in protein digestion and synthesis, carbon dioxide transport, and vitamin A utilization	Delayed wound healing; impaired taste sensitivity. Severe deficiency (in U.S.): retarded growth and sexual development; dwarfism	Oysters, herring; meat, liver; fish; milk; whole grains; nuts; legumes

Appendix C

Useful Herbs and Oils

The following are easily obtainable and might be useful in a variety of settings. Always try a small amount on a single spot to test for skin sensitivity. Talk with your health professional before using any of those that are to be taken internally.

Almond oil. Useful for therapeutic massage or as a base for other oils as in aromatherapy. It is a natural nut oil high in fatty acids. It is commonly found in creams and soaps.

Aloe vera. It is a gel obtained from the inner tissue of leaves of the aloe vera plant. It has soothing and healing qualities for the skin (e.g., can soothe a burn) and hair. It is also useful as an astringent.

Avocado oil. It comes from avocado and is useful in maintaining soft skin. It contains a number of vitamins (A,D, and E—carotenoids, phytoseral, lecithin).

Boneset. Used to relieve aches and pains of colds and flu. It has sweat-inducing properties that are useful in bringing down a fever.

Buchu leaves. Used in Europe for maintaining urinary tract health.

Calendula. Used to treat inflamed areas and is thought to promote cell formation. It is extracted from the marigold flower.

Camphor. Aids in controlling swelling of the tissues and thereby aids in providing more nutrients and oxygen with the result of more rapid healing. It is an oil found in the wood of the camphor tree.

Chamomile. Soothes the skin and mends split ends in the hair. It comes from the blossoms of the chamomile plant.

Dandelion root. It has a laxative effect and a diuretic effect; must be used carefully.

Echinacea (*Echinacea purpurea*). Useful in more rapidly decreasing the symptoms of a cold or flu. Acts as an immune system tonic.

Eucalyptus. Acts as an antiseptic and antibacterial. It comes from the leaves of the eucalyptus tree. It is also found in bath oils and therapeutic massage oils.

Evening primrose oil. Used to improve the skin (a linoleic oil) when taken internally or applied externally. It is an essential oil from the yellow evening primrose flower. Found in shampoos and hair conditioners, the oil removes tangles and repairs split ends.

Fenugreek seeds. Useful in improving gastrointestinal tract function through the soothing mucilaginous material it contains; said to have a blood sugar–lowering effect but not adequate enough to be considered a useful treatment by scientific research.

Feverfew (*Chrysanthemum parthenium*). Useful for headaches, especially in prevention of migraines. Has been found useful in the inflammatory stage of arthritis.

Garlic. Useful in lowering cholesterol levels (in the allicin form) and blood pressure. Promotes digestion by affecting the pathogenic organisms in the intestine while supporting the helpful bacteria.

Ginger. Helpful in easing nausea, flatulence, diarrhea, and dizziness. Is known to prevent nausea from morning sickness, stomach flu, and motion sickness.

Ginkgo (*Ginkgo biloba*). Supports blood flow, especially to the brain. Helpful in treating early stages of Alzheimer's disease.

Grapefruit seed (extract). Obtained from the grapefruit seed, it has antifungal and antiviral properties. It is usually mixed with other preservatives.

Hawthorn. For treating early symptoms of heart disease by increasing the blood supply to the heart.

Honey. It can be used as a natural moisturizer for the hair and skin; it helps to retain moisture.

Horsetail. Used in strengthening the hair strands. It has a high concentration of silica.

Lavender oil. Useful in soothing minor skin irritations and, in a base such as almond oil, is useful in therapeutic massage, especially for a cramped muscle or other area of discomfort. Note: there are a variety of lavender oils. The *Lavandula angustifolia* is the most common one used for massage and relief of discomfort.

Lemongrass. Useful in tightening open pores. It is also useful for nails and skin.

Milk thistle. Believed to protect and tone liver cells by strengthening liver cell membranes. Also helps to promote digestion.

Nettles. Used in hair care products to help stimulate the hair follicles and to regulate scalp oil buildup. It does have a high nutritional value (iron and potassium). It is know for its painful sting.

Oatmeal. Used to remove dry and dead skin and to unclog blocked pores in the skin. It is called an exfoliant.

Passionflower. Useful in easing muscle tension and emotional distress. Is known for inducing sleep as a natural calming agent.

Peppermint. When used in shampoos it reduces scalp flakiness, and in lotions or creams or any product, like toothpaste, for its cooling sensation. The oil of peppermint contains menthol.

Plantain. Used in soothing wounds. This plant possesses antiseptic, astringent, and styptic (assists in stopping bleeding) properties.

Raspberry leaves. A remedy for diarrhea; also useful in treating wounds.

Rosemary. Used to stimulate blood circulation to the skin and to strengthen the hair. It is an essential oil of the rosemary flower.

Rosewater. Used in soothing irritated skin. It is obtained from the extraction of rose oil, it has a honey and rose scent and is slightly antiseptic.

Sage oil. It is an anti-inflammatory that has a mild astringent and stimulating effect. It appears to aid in the healing of wounds.

Saw palmetto berries. Useful in countering enlarged prostate glands and in treating genito-urinary tract infections.

Seaweed. Contains minerals, vitamins, and amino acids. It is used for nourishing and healing the skin. It is also found in hair products.

Shea butter. Useful in moisturizing and nourishing the skin. It is obtained from the fatty substance found in the berry nut of the African karite tree. If used in large quantities it can be a protectant from the sun's rays.

St. John's wort. Useful as an astringent, an antiinflammatory, and has antibiotic properties when used on the skin. Now recognized as an antidepressant when used internally. It comes from the oils extracted from the leaves of this plant.

Tea tree oil. Useful antiseptic that is both antimicrobial and antibacterial. It comes from the leaves of the Australian melaleuca trees. It is used in skin care products for the treatment of acne, psoriasis, and other skin irritations. In shampoos and rinses, it is useful for treating flaky scalp conditions.

Valerian (*Valerlunu ufficinalis*). Uooful as a sleep inducer while easing nervous tension. It also acts as a sedative for emotional disturbances
and pain.

Vitamins A and E. Internally, these are antioxidants. Externally, they
are preservatives, preventing scaliness and dryness of the skin. These
vitamins have been found helpful in treating skin rashes and skin ulcers.
Vitamin E promotes the growth of tissue cells.

Some of the above have been adapted from the *Feather River Company
Catalog* and *Zia Cosmetic Ingredient Dictionary.*

Appendix D

Botanical Names of Common Herbs

Specific dosages, indications, and contraindications may be obtained from the *Herbal Physicians' Desk Reference* and other resources

Alfalfa (*Medicago sativa*)
Aloe (*Aloe vera*)
Artichoke (*Cynara scolymus*)
Barley (*Hordeum vulgare*)
Bilberry (*Vaccinuim myrtillus*)
Bitter melon (*Momordica charantia*)
Black cohosh (*Cimiafuga racemosa*)
Burdock root (*Arctium lappa*)
Cayenne (*Capsicum annuum*)
Cinnamon (*Cinnamomum verum*)
Coneflower, purple (*Echinacea purpurea*)
Evening primrose (*Oenothera biennis*)
Fenugreek seeds (*Trigonella foenum-graecum*)
Fo-ti (*Polygonum multiflorum*)
Garlic (*Allium sativum*)
Ginger (*Zingiber officinale*)
Ginkgo (*Ginkgo biloba*)
Ginseng (*Panax ginseng*)
Ginseng, Siberian (*Eleutherococcus senticosus*)
Green tea (*Camellia sinensis*)
Guar gum (*Camopsis tetragonolobus*)
Juniper (*Juniperus communis*)

Kava kava (*Piper methysticum*)
Psyllium seed (*Plantago afra*)
Sage (*Salvia officinales*)
Saw palmetto (*Serenoa repens*)
St. John's wort (*Hypericum perforatum*)
Yellowroot/Goldenseal (*Hydrastic canadensis*)

Appendix E

Herbs that Change Blood Glucose Levels

Herbs that Lower Blood Glucose Levels*

Aceitilla (*Bidens pilosa*)—plant
Adiantum (*Adiantum capillus-veneris*)—plant
Agrimony (*Agrimonia eupatoria*)—leaves
Akee (*Blighia sapida*)—seeds/unripened fruit
Aloe (*Aloe vera*)—gel/dried exudate
Banana (*Musa sapientum*)—flowers and roots
Banyan (*Ficus bengalensis*)—stem bark
Barleria (*Hygrophila auriculata*)—plant
Barley (*Hordeum vulgare*)—sprouts
Bilberry (*Vaccinium myrtillus*)—leaves
Bitter melon (*Momordica charantia*)—fruit
Box thorn (*Lycium barbarum*)—leaves
Bugleweed (*Lycopus virginicus*)—plant
Burdock (*Arctium lappa*)—roots
Carob (*Ceratonia siliqua*)—bean gum
Cashew (*Anacardium occidentale*)—leaves
Catarinita (*Salpianthus arenarius*)—flowers
Coccinia (*Coccina grandis*)—roots
Copalchi (*Coutarea latiflora*)—root bark
Corn (*Zea mays*)—silk stigmas
Cucumber (*Cumcumis sativus*)—fruit
Cumin (*Cuminum cyminum*)—seed
Damiana (*Turnera diffusa*)—leaves

Dandelion (*Taraxacum officinale*)—plant
Devil's club (*Fatsia herrida = Oplaopanax horridum*)—root bark
Eucalyptus (*Eucalyptus globulus*)—leaves
Fenugreek (*Trigonella foenum-graecum*)—seeds
Fluggea (*Securinega virosa*)—seeds
Fo-ti (*Polygonum multiflorum*)—root
Garlic (*Allium sativum*)—cloves
Ginseng (*Panax ginseng*)—roots
Ginseng, Siberian (*Eleutherococcus senticosus*)—root
Goat's rue (*Galega officinalis*)—seeds
Guar gum (*Camopsis tetragonolobus*)—seeds and pods
Guarumo (*Cecropia obtusifolia*)—leaves and stem
Gulacha (*Tinospora cordifolia*)—plant
Gurmar (*Gymnema sylvestre*)—leaves
Horse chestnuts (*Aeculus hippocastanum*)—seeds
Injerto flowers (*Psittacanthus calyuculatus*)—leaves and stem
Ivy gourd (*Coccinia indica*)—leaves
Jambul (*Syzygium cumini*)—seeds
Juniper berries (*Juniperus communis*)
Jute (*Corchorus olitorius*)—leaves
Kidney bean (*Phaseolus vulgaris*)—immature pods
Konjak tubers (*Amorphophallus knojac*)—tubers
Lagerstroemia (*Lagerstroemia speciosa*)—leaves and fruit
Lotus (*Nymphaea lotus*)—roots
Lupine (*Lupinus albus*)—seeds
Madagascar periwinkle (*Vinca rosea*)—leaves
Maitake mushroom (*Grifola frondosa*)—the mushroom body
Mulberry (*Morus alba*)—leaves
Olive (*Olea europaea*)—leaves
Onion (*Allium cepa*)—bulbs
Phyllanthus (*Phyllanthus niruri*)—leaves
Prickly pear (*Opuntia*)—cactus plant
Psyllium (*Plantago psyllium*)—seed
Reishi mushroom (*Ganoderma lucidum*)—the mushroom body
Rivea (*Argyreia cuneata*)—leaves
Sacred basil (*Ocimum sanctum*)—plant
Salt bush (*Atriplex halimus*)—leaves
Solomon's seal (*Polygonatum multiflorum*)—root
Spinach (*Spinaceal oleracea*)—leaves
Staghorn sumac (*Rhus typina*)—leaves
Sweet broom (*Scorparia dulcis*)—plant

Thornay burnet (*Sarcopoterium spinosum*)—root bark
Tronador (*Tecoma stans*)—leaves
Wheat (*Triticum sativum*)—leaves
White button mushroom (*Agaricus bisporus*)—the mushroom body
White lupine (*Lupinus albus*)—seeds
White mulberry (*Morus alba*)—leaves
Willowstrife (*Lythrum salicaria*)—plant

Herbs that Raise Blood Glucose Levels*

Annatto (*Bixa orellana*)—seeds
Cocoa (*Theobroma cacao*)—seeds
Coffee (*Coffea arabica*)—seeds
Cola (*Cola acuminata*)—seeds
Guarana (*Paullinia cupana*)—seeds
Mahuang (*Ephedra sinica*)—plant
Maté (*Ilex paraguayensis*)—leaves
Rosemary (*Rosmarinus officinalis*)—leaves
Tea (*Camellia sinensis*)—leaves

---

*For more information read Francis Brinker's book *Herb Contraindications and Drug Interactions,* 2nd ed. Eclectic Medical Publications, Sandy, Oregon, 1998.

APPENDIX F

RESOURCE NAMES AND ADDRESSES

Academy for Guided Imagery, P.O. Box 2070, Mill Valley, CA 94942; 800-726-2070

American Botanical Council, P.O. Box 144345, Austin, TX 78714-4345

American Diabetes Association, 1701 N. Beauregard St., Alexander, VA 22311; 800-232-3472

American Dietetics Association, 216 W. Jackson Blvd., Chicago, IL 60606-1600; 800-877-1600

American Herbalists Guild, P.O. Box 70, Roosevelt, UT 84066; 435-722-8434

American Herbal Pharmacopoeia, P.O. Box 5159, Santa Cruz, CA 05063; 408-461-6317

American Herbal Products Association; 512-469-6355

American Holistic Nurses Association, P.O. Box 2130, Flagstaff, AZ 86003-2130; 800-278-2462

American Sleep Disorders Association, 1610 Fourteenth St. NW, Suite 300, Rochester, MN 55901; 507-287-6006

Association for Applied Psychophysiology & Biofeedback, 10200 W. Forty-fourth Ave., Suite 304, Wheat Ridge, CO 80033; 303-422-8436

Biofeedback Institute, 3428 Sacramento Street, San Francisco, CA 94118

Institute for Safe Medication Practices; 800-324-5723

International Healing Touch Association, 198 Union Blvd., Suite 210, Lakewood, CO 89228; 303-090-0581

National Center for Complementary and Alternative Clearinghouse, P.O. Box 8218, Silver Springs, MD 20907-8218; 888-644-6226.

NIH National Center for Complementary and Alternative Medicine, 9000 Rockville Pike, Mailstop 2182, Bldg. 31, Rm. 5B-38 Bethesda, MD 20892; 301-435-5042 for professional assistance

Office of Disease Prevention & Health Promotion, National Health Information Center, P.O. Box 1133, Washington, DC 20013-1133; 800-336-4797

Professional Nurse Healers Association International, 11250 Roger Bacon Dr., Suite #8, Reston, VA 20190-5202; 703-437-4377

US Pharmacopoeia, 12601 Twinbrook Pkwy, Rockville, MD 20852; 301-881-0666

APPENDIX G

WEB SITES

Alternative Nature Online Herbal and Photo Gallery	*www.altnature.com*
American Association of Clinical Endocrinologists (AACE)	*www.aace.com*
American Association of Diabetes Educators (AADE)	*www.aadenet.org*
American Association of Medical Acupuncturists	*www.medicalacupuncture.org*
American Association of Osteopaths	*www.aao.medguide.net*
American Botanical Council (ABC)	*www.herbalgram.org*
American Chiropractic Association (ACA)	*www.amerchiro.org*
American Diabetes Association (ADA)	*www.diabetes.org*
American Dietetic Association (AdiA)	*www.webmaster@eatright.org*
American Herbalist Guild (AHG)	*www.healthy.net*
American Holistic Medical Association (AHMA)	*www.ahmaholistic.com*
American Holistic Nurses Association (AHNA)	*www.ahna.org*
American Massage Therapy Association (AMTA)	*www.amtamassage.org*
American Naturopathic Association (AANP)	*www.naturopathic.org*
Apothe'Cure	*www.apothecure.com*
Biofeedback Certification Institute of America (BCIA)	*www.bcia.org*

BMI calculations | *www.shapeup.org*
Center for Complementary | *www.camra.ucdavis.edu*
and Alternative Medicine
Centers for Disease Control | *www.cdc.gov/nccdphp/ddt/ddthome*
Diabetes Home Page
Children with Diabetes (CD) | *www.childrenwithdiabetes.com*
Diabetes Course (graduate level) | *www.feist.com/~dguthrie*
Dietary Guidelines | *www.na/usda.gov/fnic.dga/*
dguide95.html

General Diabetes Information | *www.diabetesworld.com*
Healing Touch International (HTI) | *www.healingtouch.net*
Health Information | *www.healthy.net4*
Health on the Net Foundation | *www.sympatico.ca/healthyway*
(HON)
Insulin Management | *www.insulin.org/managing/*
discussion.html

Juvenile Diabetes Foundation | *www.jdfcure.org*
(JDF)
Meal Plans Personalized | *www.healthyideas.com*
Medical Herbalism | *http://medherb.com*
National Center for | *www.nccam.nih.gov*
Complementary and
Alternative Medicine

National Institute of Diabetes, | *www.niddk.nih.gov/NIDDK_Homepage*
Digestive and Kidney
Disorders
National Institute of Health | *http://dietary-suplements.info.nih.gov*
Dietary Information
Natural Health Line | *www.naturalhealthline.com*
North American Society | *www.homeopathy.org/nash*
of Homeopaths (NASH)
PhytoPharmica | *www.phytopharmica.com*
President of the American College | *www.drjanson.com*
of Alternative Medicine
Professional Nurse Healers | *www.therapeutic-touch.org*
Quackwatch | *www.quackwatch.com*
Special Nutritional Adverse Event | *http://cfsan.fda.gov/~dms/aems.html*
Monitoring System
Spectrapham Online | *www.ruhealthy.com*
United States Pharmacopia (USP) | *www.usp.org*

Glossary

Types of Therapy

Allopathic or **orthodox medicine**   the traditional or modern medicine and the most common type of medicine used in the United States.

Alternative medicine   not scientifically based, this approach to care is used in place of allopathic medicine.

Aromatherapy   the use of herbal medicine by the administration of the medicinal properties found in the essential oils of various plants (i.e., antibacterial, antiviral, antispasmodic, diuretic, vasodilators, vasoconstrictors, immune system modifiers, and as harmonizers of moods and emotions).

Ayurvedic medicine   the approach to the overall health profile of an individual that identifies a person's constitution through metabolic body type (*doshas*): *vata* (unpredictable, slender), *pitta* (predictable, medium build), or *kapha* (relaxed, heavy build). A specific treatment plan is then designed to guide the individual back into harmony through the alteration of diet, exercise, yoga, medication, etc. (Call 619-551-7788 or www.chopra.com for information on the Chopra Center for Well-Being.)

Barbara Brennan Healing Science   this is a hands-on technique to reorganize and revitalize the client's energy field. Barbara Brennen is known as a healer and teacher with credentials as a physicist.

Chelation therapy   from *chele* (to bind) and to get rid of unnecessary and toxic metals usually through the intravenous administration of specific fluids (sometimes done with enemas). There is a specific technique in healing touch called chelation therapy whose purpose is to rid the body of energy blockages.

Chinese herbal medicine   three-thousand-year-old use of herbs in relation to five elements, and yin and yang flow.

Chiropractic medicine   drugless use of manipulation to align the spine and bones to promote the activity of nerve impulses. Chiropractic medicine attempts to alter and thereby harmonize the relationship of the spinal column and the musculoskeletal structures of the body to the nervous system so that the body may better heal itself.

Complementary medicine   may not be scientifically based, but used in addition to allopathic care.

Herbal medicine   the use of plants for healing purposes.

Homeopathic medicine   based on the system of like cures like; started in the 1800s.

Naturopathic medicine   drugless therapy based on the body's ability to heal itself.

Naturopathic therapy   an array of healing practices that include clinical nutrition, homeopathy, acupuncture, herbal medicine, hydrotherapy, therapeutic exercise, manipulation, use of electric currents, ultrasound, light therapy, therapeutic counseling, and pharmacology. This is done by treating the whole person's cause rather that the effect and facilitating the power of nature.

Osteopathic medicine   the physical medicine that helps restore the structural balance of the musculoskeletal system. This involves joint manipulation, physical therapy, and postural reeducation.

Shamanism   found in almost every culture and used for thousands and thousands of years in calling upon the spirit world for guidance in healing or curing the subject.

Natural and Holistic Healing

Acupuncture   the stimulation along twelve major pathways called meridians (over one thousand points) to balance the flow of *chi* or vital energy. (Acupressure is when external pressure is applied to one of these points.)

Colon therapy   the use of a series of water flushes to clean or "detoxify" the lower intestine and aid in the constitution of the intestinal flow.

Craniosacral therapy   a method of palpation of the motion of craniosacral system and thereby assisting the return of the balance of the cerebrospinal fluid to a unified integrated movement. This is accomplished through the manipulation of the sutures of the skull or through the manipulation of the meninges (underlying membranes) or by the stimulation of the nerve endings in the scalp.

Cupping   performed through the use of suction as a result of heating the air in a cup and placing it on areas of the skin that need the circulation improved and/or the discomfort lessened.

Herbal therapy   the use of herbs (leaf, flower, stem, seed, root, fruit, bark) for the fragrance, medicinal properties, or flavoring, to aid in altering various health conditions (i.e., from the mild-acting medicines such as chamomile to potent medication such as digitalis (foxglove).

Herbal Language

Cold maceration	placed in water for eight, plus or minus, hours.
Decoction	heated (about eight minutes) and strained.
Extract	concentrated powder or liquid from the dried plant part (leaves and/or flower and/or root).
Infusion	steeped (about eight minutes) in boiling water.
Plant juice	water-soaked and pressed fresh plants.
Standardized	pure product and/or same amount per dose (per capsule or tablet; per dose of tincture or extract).
Teas	placed in a drinkable form.
Tincture	placed in alcohol solution.
Volatile oils	distilled from crude drug.

Moxibustion   the use of burning dried mugwort to increase the flow of energy usually to a specific site.

Nutraceuticals   any substance that may be considered a food, or a part of a food, that provides medical or health benefits, including the prevention and treatment of disease such as genetically engineered "designer" foods, herbal products, dietary supplements, and isolated nutrients.

Nutrition   the choice, source, and amounts of food eaten to support adequate growth, support immune function, and promote freedom of ingestion of toxic food substances.

Bodywork, Energy, and Movement Techniques

Acupressure   the pressing on specific points on the body (twelve pathways or meridians—for over one thousand points) to relieve certain ailments by releasing energy blocks in the meridians (Acu-Yoga uses the whole body while Do-In uses body awareness through stretching and breathing and thereby affecting these more than one thousand points).

Alexander technique   the alteration of faulty posture in sitting, standing, and moving to connect with physical and emotional problems through rebalancing the body.

Feldenkrais method   the use of self-image to bring about change in one's mode of action through the use of breathing, proper movement, awareness, and through hands-on functional integration.

Hellerwork   the use of combining deep touch and movement education (from the Rolfing method) with verbal dialogue in order to facilitate an awareness of the body-mind relationship.

Jin Shin Jyutsu   an Asian therapy to harmonize the energy flow of the body. Although it involves manipulation of the muscles and pressure on the pulses by the hands, its purpose is to restore balance and thereby reduce stress.

Myotherapy (or **Bonnie Prudden technique**)   using the elbow or fingers to pressure the areas affected with spasms and other discomfort.

Reflexology   the stimulation of reflexes through pressure and massage of various areas of the hands and feet that correspond to every part of the body. This is used to relieve tension, promote relaxation, improve circulation, and promote the unblocking of nerve impulses in order to rebalance the body.

Reiki   an energy therapy with the purpose of supporting the body's healing process through the placement of hands in corresponding positions and the use of symbols in order to allow a flow of energy through that body part.

Rolfing   the massage of deep tissues. Also called Structural Integration.

Rosen method   a questioning process while the person is receiving deep but gentle pressure especially on tense muscles.

Shiatsu   a massage method based on the meridian acupuncture points. It is believed to promote healing as well as relax the subject.

Sports massage   muscle kneading and range of motion are focused on relieving pain and promoting relaxation.

Swedish massage   a method of massage using forty-seven positions and over eight hundred movements to relieve muscle tension, increase muscle tone, increase muscle balance, and for general relaxation. The five major strokes are effleurage (stroking), petrissage (kneading), friction (rocking), tapotement (percussion), and vibration (by machine or hand).

Tae-Bo   a combination of martial arts and anaerobic sequencing of activity usually accompanied by rhythmic music.

Therapeutic touch   the conscious effort to draw upon energy for healing purposes. This generally requires a variety of physical to non-physical contact through the process of centering, assessing, unruffling, modulation, and smoothing (and reassessing). It has been used to enhance healing, relieve pain, help relaxation, and reduce inflammation.

Yoga   the union of the physical, mental, and spiritual energies that enhance health and well-being through physical postures to promote the even flow of *prana* or energy throughout the body.

Counseling

Art therapy   for treating emotional and behavioral problems.

Biofeedback   the use of information obtained through temperature, electromyography, pulse rate, galvanic skin response, or other body information that indicates a learning or relearning of body processes. The training is used to learn how to consciously change or regulate unconscious body functions in order to decrease pain or increase movement.

Hypnotherapy   the use of suggestion to effect positive changes in a person's behavior through the induction of a deep level of relaxation. Its major use is to enhance the mind's contribution to healing.

Music therapy   the use of sound and music to slow the breathing and/or the heart rate or influence other bodily functions, to create a feeling of well-being, and to support relaxation.

Normal Laboratory Values

Note: values may be somewhat higher or lower for your particular hospital or clinic, depending on the method used to run the tests.

Alkaline phosphatase	30–85 ImU/ml (up to 300 in children)
BUN	5–20 mg/dl
Calcium	9.0–10.5 mg/dl
Chloride	90–110 mEq/L
CO_2	23–30 mEq/L
Creatinine	less than 1.4 mg/dl females and 1.5 mg/dl males
Glucose	70–110 mg/dl (FPG)
Hematocrit	37–52%
Hemoglobin A_{1c}	4.3–6.7 (varies with laboratory)
Magnesium	1.6–3.0 mEq/L

Phosphorous	2.5–4.5 mg/dl
Potassium	3.5–5.0 mEq/L
SGPT (ALT)	5–35 IU/L
SGOT (AST)	12–36 IU/L
Sodium	136–145 mEq/L

BIBLIOGRAPHY

These are just some of the available books in print.

Albright, P. *The Complete Book of Complementary Therapies: The Best-Known Alternative Therapies to Relieve Everyday Ailments.* Allentown, Pa.: People's Medical Society, 1997. This colorful and brightly illustrated book is written by a physician. The chapter on diabetes includes, as for other ailments, short, research-based statements, in most part, of supportive therapy.

Aspen Reference Group. *Holistic Health Promotion and Complementary Therapies: A Resource for Integrated Practice.* Gaithersburg, Md.: Aspen Publishers, 1998. This professional resource includes foundations for the field; a focus on various modalities; guidelines for application and use for common human problems, and planning strategies to develop integrative practices.

Balch, J. E. and P. A. Balch. *Prescription for Nutritional Healing,* 2nd ed. Garden City Park, N.Y.: Avery Publishing Group, 1997. Organized by disease and by condition or problem, it includes overview on each plus general information on nutrition, vitamin and minerals, and charts on associated nutrients and suggested dosages. For each disease or problem, recommendations are made for herbs and why they should be considered of use.

Barney, D. P. *Clinical Applications of Herbal Medicine.* Pleasant Groove, Utah: Woodland Publishing, 1996. This physician describes the use of herbs for a variety of specific conditions and illnesses. A chapter is devoted to diabetes and also to low blood sugar. Amounts of herbs in the recommended formula are not included, so careful guidance is needed when determining the use of such combinations.

Bratman, S. *The Alternative Medicine Sourcebook: A Realistic Evaluation of Alternatives.* Los Angeles: Lowell House, 1998. A basic guide for finding a qualified practitioner, learning the strengths and weaknesses of alternative approaches, integrating conventional and alternative medicine, and treating common illnesses.

Benson, H. and E. M. Stuart. *The Wellness Book: The Comprehensive Guide to Maintaining Health and Treating Stress-Related Illness.* New York: Simon & Schuster, 1993. By the same author as *The Relaxation Response,* this book includes a number of topics specifically related to diabetes. Workbook-type activities are spaced throughout the narrative from a self-esteem checklist to a humor commitment worksheet.

Besset, N. G., ed. *Max Wichtl Herbal Drugs and Phytopharmaceuticals: A Handbook for Practice on a Scientific Basis.* Ann Arbor, Mich.: Medpharm Scientific Publishers, 1994. A very informative, international text that contains illustrations, indications, and side effects of 181 herbs.

Brennan, B. A. *Hands Of Light: A Guide to Healing through the Human Energy Field.* New York: Bantam Books, 1997. Includes an excellent description of the human energy fields and the quantum physics associated with energy therapy. It also relates self-care techniques and considerations for personal growth.

Brigham, D. D. *Imagery for Getting Well: Clinical Applications of Behavioral Medicine.* New York: W. W. Norton & Company, 1994. It includes different approaches to the use of imagery in various situations. Imagery is also associated with the use of other modalities including therapeutic touch and Qigong.

Brinker, F. *Herb Contraindications and Drug Interactions: With Appendices Addressing Specific Conditions and Medicines,* 2nd ed. Sandy, Oreg.: Eclectic Medical Publications, 1998. Reviews herbs to be used with caution; herb/drug interactions; herbs contraindicated for pregnant women and children; and vitamin/mineral/drug interactions.

Buckle, J. *Clinical Aromatherapy in Nursing.* San Diego, Cal.: Singular Publishing Group, 1997. This very informative book was specifically written for nurses, but the reader will receive useful information on the field and its uses and a greater appreciation of Florence Nightingale, a nurse who was quite ahead of her time.

Burton Goldberg Group, eds. *Alternative Medicine: The Definitive Guide.* Puyallup, Wash.: Future Medicine Publishing, 1994. An easily readable resource for health professional and lay person alike. It includes all the major therapies and many of the minor ones in clear and concise language.

Callahan R. J. and J. Callahan. *Thought Field Therapy (TFT) and Trauma: Treatment and Theory.* Indian Wells, Cal.: TFT Training Center, 1996. This book is an overview of the field of (TFT), especially in the treatment of post-traumatic stress disorders. It introduces the terms and simple techniques that can be of assistance to the practitioner.

Cassileth, B. *The Alternative Medicine Handbook: The Complete Reference Guide to Alternative and Complementary Therapies.* New York: W. W. Norton & Company, 1998. The author was a founding member of the Advisory Council to the National Institutes of Health Office of Alternative Medicine. She includes material on spiritual, emotional, dietary, herbal, alternative biological treatments, use of external energy forces, and the reduction of pain and stress through body work. Also useful is a listing of complementary therapies for some common ailments. Diabetes is mentioned on a number of pages.

Chopra, D. *Quantum Healing.* New York: Bantam, 1989. The physics behind it all is the central theme of this book. It also includes the description of the body types and recommendations for their health and healing (one of his earliest publications).

Colbin, A. *Food and Healing: How What You Eat Determines Your Health, Your Well-Being, and the Quality of Your Life.* New York: Ballantine Books, 1996. Reviews a number of types of diets and how food can be used as "medicine."

Dollemore, D., M. Guiliucci, J. Haigh, S. Kirchheimer, and J. Callahan. *New Choices in Natural Healing: Over 1,800 of the Best Self-Help Remedies from the World of Alternative Medicine.* Emmaus, Pa.: Rodale Press, 1995. As it states, by disease or by therapy, much information which is condensed into short paragraphs.

Dossey, L. *Prayer Is Good Medicine: How to Reap the Healing Benefits of Prayer.* San Francisco: HarperCollins, 1996. Useful as a resource for information concerning research on prayer and suggestions on including prayer in your lifestyle or more effective praying ideas if prayer is part of your daily activity.

Duke, J. A. *The Green Pharmacy.* New York: St. Martin's Press, 1997. This is a compendium of natural remedies indexed according to health problems. It gives a good recipe for Dia-Beanie Soup along with information from authorities in the field.

Firshein, R. *The Nutraceutical Revolution: 20 Cutting-Edge Nutrients to Help You Design Your Own Perfect Whole-Life Program.* New York: Penguin Putnam, Inc., 1998. The author is an osteopath who has reviewed the literature and comments in depth on the most common nutrients found in grocery stores and health food stores.

Foster, S. and V. E. Tyler. *The Honest Herbal.* Pharmaceutical Products Press, 1999. This is a useful resource when trying to determine if an herb is useful and if it is safe. Guidance is given in relation to ways of determining if a specific herb chosen is a safe one to use.

Fugh-Berman, A. *Alternative Medicine: What Works.* Baltimore, Md.: Williams & Wilkins Publishers, 1997. This is, as is stated, "a comprehensive, easy-to-read review of the scientific evidence, pro and con" of alternative medicine. Specifically for the public, it defines the terms associated with research and reviews a variety of groups of modalities used in this practice.

Hale, T. *The Hale Clinic: Guide to Good Health: How to Choose the Right Alternative Therapy.* Woodstock, N.Y.: Overlook Press, 1997. A focus on various health problems rather than on diseases, what is done by the orthodox approach and what is done by the Hale approach, beautifully illustrated by colored photographs. The Hale approach includes the use of alternative and complementary modalities that have been useful for that specific problem.

Hoffman, J. *Rhythmic Medicine: Music with a Purpose.* Leawood, Kans.: Jamillan Press, 1995. This book is a must for guidance in using music as therapy. Enclosed is an order blank for types of music to fit various emotional needs.

Huang, K. C. *The Pharmacology of Chinese Herbs,* 2nd ed. New York: CRC Press, 1999. This book describes the chemistry, actions, and therapeutic use of various herbs used in traditional Chinese medicine. Its appendix contains a list of Chinese equivalents of the names of herbs.

Jackson, M. and T. Teague. *The Handbook of Alternative to Chemical Medicine.* Novato, Cal.: New World Library, 1997. Written by two doctors of naturopathy, this information should contribute to your discussions with health-care providers when considering treatment and emergency care for common complaints. Its appendixes include a guide for the uses and sources for various vitamins and minerals.

Joy, W. B. *Joy's Way: A Map for the Transformational Journey.* Los Angeles: Jeremy P. Tarcher, 1979. A classic introduction to the potentials for healing with body energies. At this time of the eleventh anniversary edition, it describes the major energy fields and their importance.

Katzman, S. and W. Shankin-Cohen. *Feeling Light: The Holistic Solution to Permanent Weight Loss and Wellness.* New York: Avon Books, 1997. This is a guide for changing your way of life. The chapter on the cleansing fast is not for people with Type 1 diabetes unless it is carefully coordinated with a health professional.

Kirschmann, G. J. and J. D. Kirschmann. *Nutrition Almanac,* 4th ed. New York: McGraw-Hill, 1996. Organized by disease entities and vitamin and mineral deficiencies, it offers a synopsis of the disease plus a listing of nutrients that might be beneficial in the treatment of the problem.

Macrae, J. *Therapeutic Touch: A Practical Guide.* New York: Alfred A. Knopf Publishers, 1987. This is a basic guide on learning therapeutic touch. It also includes suggestions on how to incorporate TT in daily life. (Other books on TT are also available from the 1990s.)

Mannion, M. *354 Everyday Health Tips: A Daily Guide to Improving Health and Increasing Energy.* Baltimore, Md.: Ottenheimer Publishers, 1996. This book is full of useful suggestions for improving everyday self-care.

Matthews, D. A. *The Faith Factor: Proof of the Healing Power of Prayer.* New York: Viking, 1998. The name says it all. This physician reviews the science, discusses spirituality, and combines these two areas of information in the final section of the book.

Mitchell, D. R. *Natural Medicine for Diabetes: A Comprehensive, Up-To-Date Guide to Complementary, Drug-Free Therapies.* New York: Lynn Sonberg, 1997. This paperback book includes therapy recommendations to promote circulation and to control blood glucose levels, dietary guidelines, and the use of common herbs for healing.

Mitchell, S. *Massage: A Step-by-Step Aproach to the Healing Art of Touch.* Boston: Element, 1997. This book deals with aromatherapy, shiatsu, hydrotherapy, reflexology, and inversion therapy.

Murray, M. T. *The Healing Power of Herbs: The Enlightened Person's Guide to the Wonder of Medicinal Plants.* 2nd ed. Rocklin, Cal.: Prima Publishing, 1995. Each herb identified is accompanied by a general description, its chemical composition, the history of its use, its pharmacology, dosages, toxicology, and references.

Rapgay, L. *The Tibetan Book of Healing.* Salt Lake City: Passage Press, 1998. The first conference on this type of healing in the United States was held in the fall of 1998. From diagnosis through to the use of therapeutics, this book describes a variety of modalities, some of which are not noted in other practices.

Rosenfeld, I. *Doctor, What Should I Eat?* New York: Random House, 1995. Written by a physician, it includes recommendations for eating related to a variety of illnesses and conditions. There is a separate chapter on diabetes and dietary needs.

Ryan, R. S. and J. W. Travis. *Wellness: Small Changes You Can Use to Make a Big Difference.* Berkeley, Cal.: Ten Speed Press, 1991. An informative and useful tool combining complementary and traditional practices for good health care.

Sadler, J. *Natural Pain Relief: A Practical Handbook for Self-Help.* Rockport, Mass.: Element, 1997. Guidance in the use of relaxation practices, enhancing self-esteem, and dealing with feelings that form the basis for useful suggestions to deal with chronic pain.

Teegarden, I. M. *A Complete Guide to Acupressure.* Japan Publications, 1996. A useful, up-to-date reference book.

Weil, A. *Spontaneous Healing.* New York: Alfred A. Knopf, 1995. A physician's view of healing through optimal nutrition. It includes an eight-week plan for diet, supplements, exercise, and mental/spiritual growth.

Weiss, R. J., G. Subak-Sharpe, and the Editors of the Consumer Reports Books. *40+ Guide to Good Health.* Yonkers, N.Y.: Consumer Reports Books, 1993. Includes needs for lifestyle changes of good health, stress reduction methods, exercise program suggestions, research on preventing heart disease, and strategies for "lifelong mental and emotional fitness."

Williams, R. J. *The Wonderful World within You: Understanding Your Individual Differences Can Be the Key to a Healthier, More Vigorous Life.* Wichita, Kans.: Bio-Communication Press, 1998. Foods are composed of a variety of carbohydrate, protein, fat, vitamins, minerals, fiber, and fluid. This classic aids a person in choosing nutrition specific for the individual's needs.

Yang, J. M. *Eight Simple Qigong Exercises for Health,* 2nd ed. Roslindale, Mass.: YMAA Publications Center, 1997. A detailed guide for practicing Tai chi and Qigong.

Ziyin, S. and C. Zelin. *The Basis of Traditional Chinese Medicine.* Boston: Shambhala Publications, 1994. A useful book to learn more about the history and development of this type of medicine. It instructs on the yin-yang use, the five elements, and the relationship between these two. It also includes the principles of treatment and specific modalities that are related.

INDEX

Page numbers in italics refer to quotations.